Cancer Was Not a Gift & It Didn't Make Me a Better Person

A memoir about cancer as I know it

Nancy Stordahl

Also by Nancy Stordahl

Getting Past the Fear: A Guide to Help You Mentally Prepare for Chemotherapy

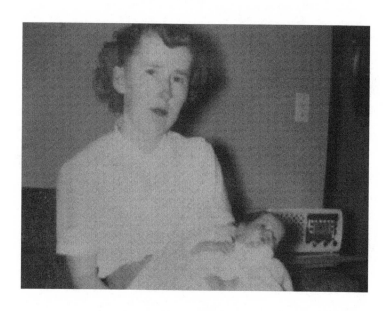

For my mother

I had known the pain, and survived it. It only remained for me to give it voice, to share it for use, that the pain not be wasted.

Audre Lorde

Acknowledgments

Thank you to my family for supporting me in my writing and non-writing endeavors. This book took five years to finish, and you never lost faith in me or doubted it would be finished. Thank you to my medical team for providing me with excellent care for the past five years. Special thanks to Dr. Chris Hower, my general surgeon; to Dr. Gopakumar S. Nambudiri, my first oncologist; to Dr. Sandeep Basu, my oncologist these days; and to Dr. James C. Banich, my plastic surgeon. Many thanks to all the fabulous nurses who took care of me as well. Thank you to my loyal readers at www.NancysPoint.com for encouraging and inspiring me every day and also to my many online friends who do the same. A huge thank you to my wonderful, patient and exceptionally skilled editor, Lindsay Stordahl. Above all, thank you to David for standing by me through the chaos of cancer and its aftermath, for knowing me so well, loving me anyway and for reminding me more than once I need no one's permission to share my story.

Disclaimer

In sharing my story it is not my intention to judge others or speak for anyone else. Everyone has the right to do, reflect upon and talk about their cancer experience in any way they choose. Within these pages are some of my cancer truths about my experience. Some of them may or may not be yours as well. In order to protect privacy, some names have been changed. All details are shared as accurately as possible and events of the past are shared to the best of my recollection. In addition, no material presented in this book is intended to replace or be interpreted in any manner as professional medical advice.

Introduction

Many body parts come in pairs and are actually far more vital to our function and well-being than breasts. When you think about it, eyes, ears, arms, legs and other body part pairs are way more important to quality of life and our ability to live and move around. But it's breasts American society is obsessed with. Women go to great lengths to make them appear bigger and sometimes smaller. We wear uncomfortable bras, some with wires that pinch, and others with cumbersome push-up pads. We buy creams, ointments and various exercise contraptions to enhance our silhouettes. We worry that our breasts are too big, too small or too saggy. Many of us undergo surgeries to make our breasts bigger or sometimes smaller. From the moment puberty hits, breasts are either powerful assets to display and flaunt, or body parts we'd rather conceal and cover up.

I discovered at an early age what powerful components of female anatomy breasts are. One of my earliest recollections of childhood is running around the house my family lived in on Central Avenue North on hot summer nights wearing only my underwear, the bottom half, of course. We lived on Central Avenue North for the first half of my childhood, and for the second half we moved to the other end of town, same street except Central Avenue South. The upstairs bedroom I shared with one of my sisters in that creaky old house we rented was incredibly hot in the summer and likewise drafty and cold in the winter. On hot, humid summer evenings I ran around minimally clothed feeling totally uninhibited and carefree, concerned only about staying cool and comfortable. Then suddenly I reached a certain age when running around in only my underwear became unacceptable. Budding breasts were undoubtedly the reason for the unstated but nonetheless explicitly known new restrictions. Modesty and being proper were suddenly more important than comfort and freedom.

A bit later when I was in fourth grade, one of my classmates abruptly and unexpectedly hit puberty and suddenly, overnight it seemed to the rest of us, she had breasts, and substantially sized ones at that. Immediately, she became someone of mystery and intrigue to those of us who had yet to blossom. With breasts she was someone to be in awe of, and the rest of us tried to look inconspicuous with our stares and sideways glances. Sadly, I remember some girls treating her badly, teasing with mean, crude remarks sometimes directly to her face, but more often behind her back. And the boys definitely noticed, especially older ones waiting to prey on inexperienced and vulnerable new targets. Yes, even at such tender, young ages we were all well aware of the almost mystical power of breasts. The girls eagerly waited for, but also dreaded the inevitable transformation of our bodies, and the boys, well, they just acted like boys and waited for their own transformations as well.

Later on, like many teenagers, I wasn't entirely happy with my new, emerging shape. I always felt a bit small in the bosom and a few times stuffed my bra with Kleenex for a little oomph. That worked fine until I started going steady and couldn't fool my boyfriend's groping hands with Kleenex.

In college I even went so far as to secretly order a "bust enhancing" exercise contraption I discovered in a magazine. The ad promised to significantly increase my measurements if I followed the directions for mere minutes a day. The device was a piece of pink plastic with a tight spring of some sort in the middle. You held the device in front of you and squeezed the two sides together. I stood in my dorm room with the door tightly shut squeezing away, but I never noticed anything happening, except for a growing realization I had been duped.

Shortly after graduating from college, my high school sweetheart David and I got married, and I came to accept my body, at least most of the time. I became confident, comfortable and just plain more mature about how I looked at myself. The days of wanting to change my body were over, well, mostly over. Later came three babies, and I proudly breastfed all three. Suddenly, my breasts were truly functioning as nature intended, and I grew to appreciate them during that special time (except for the sore nipples and painful case of mastitis). After that period, I didn't think much about breasts. Life was just too busy. Years passed and mammograms entered into my now more mature routine. I patted myself on the back for entering this new watchdog phase of breast awareness.

Then one day, out of the blue it seemed, my mother was diagnosed with breast cancer, and suddenly breasts were back in life's spotlight, now as potential betrayers and messengers of doom. After her diagnosis and death four years later from the wretched disease, I naively believed I could not be stricken for at least a while. Some reasonable period of time would have to pass. No family could be inflicted with back-to-back cancers. That would be too cruel. There must be quotas on misery allotments. Surely I would be spared, or at least given a fair amount of time to prepare. I was wrong. Cancer sticks to its own protocol, which means it doesn't follow any. It strikes whenever it damn pleases. My cancer diagnosis came in April 2010, and my personal cancer domino effect was set in motion. It continues to this day.

A few weeks later on an ordinary day in late spring, or early summer, depending on your seasonal vantage point, I said goodbye to my breasts. I miss them. I miss a lot of things about my pre-cancer life. This does not mean I'm trying to rewind my life. I'm not. My life now is good, very good. I have much to be grateful for and I am, but cancer changes everything. It just does. Cancer is a string of losses, and I will *certainly never be calling it a gift*. And just for the record, *it didn't make me a better person either.*

Within these pages, I share about cancer as I know it. I share from a daughter's perspective as a caregiver. I share about loss, my own cancer experience and some things I've learned along the way. I share about these things hoping to encourage others going through similar trials and to remind readers there is no right way to "do" cancer or grief. I share because sharing is healing, empowering and hopefully helps us all feel less alone. I share because everyone's story matters, mine, and yours, too.

-1-

I Think I'm Having a Heart Attack!

As I stand awkwardly in front of the registration desk at my local hospital under the sign displaying the words *Urgent Care*, the receptionist sitting behind the counter takes a phone call, busily sorts files and simultaneously types in information on her keyboard, hardly taking time to glance up at me. I feel as if I'm intruding. When she finally looks up, her eyes do a quick scan of my body as if she does her own kind of diagnosis each time she checks in a new patient from her secret place of power behind the counter.

"Can I help you?" she asks.

"I think I might be having a heart attack or something; I'm having chest pain," I say.

I tell her this matter-of-factly, as if I am checking in due to a sore throat or ear infection.

The words even sound ridiculous and impossible hanging in the air as they leave my lips. People my age don't have heart attacks. I look around to see if anyone else might have heard me say such unbelievable words. No one seems to have noticed.

Minutes later I am hooked up to an EKG machine in triage room #3 behind a blue curtain. When you tell someone in a hospital you think you might be having a heart attack, you bypass urgent care and get routed directly to the ER.

"It's normal, you are not having a heart attack," a nurse informs me a few minutes later, and I breathe a little more easily, unaware this is the last piece of good news I will receive today.

A little while later the ER doctor enters the room looking like he is in a hurry. He is tall, about my age, has curly, gray hair and speaks with an accent of some sort. He pulls up a stool and listens as I describe in detail how I thought I pulled a chest muscle raking piles of matted, dead leaves from my flower beds a couple weeks ago, dismissed it for a while, but finally ended up here. He studies and observes me while trying to piece together his latest patient's symptoms into some kind of neat compartment he can label. I feel as if I'm trying to convince him my story is plausible. Maybe it isn't. I'm not even sure anymore.

"It sounds like you probably did just overdo it raking and pulled a chest muscle," he says. "But we'll run some blood tests just to rule things out."

"Ruling things out is always a good idea," I say.

He gets up to leave while joking around and holding his back, pretending to have back pain.

"See, I have aches and pains too. It happens at our age," he says as he leaves the room smiling.

Now I'm starting to feel a little silly and begin to contemplate the cost of lying in an ER room all afternoon. Dollar signs and copayment costs start flashing through my mind.

After a half-dozen or so vials of blood are drawn and then analyzed by people invisible to me down the hall, the doctor returns, this time appearing slightly less jovial.

"One of your tests reveals a marker level indicating a possible blood clot in your lung. Of course, this is *extremely* unlikely," he says. "But our protocol requires me to order a CT scan, just to be sure. We are *still* simply ruling things out. Don't you worry."

This time he pats my leg as he leaves, appearing to suddenly take me a little more seriously, but just a little.

Next, I am wheeled into the CT scan room which feels frigidly cold, and I immediately start shaking from fear as much as the temperature. There is even a thermometer on the wall to closely monitor the room's temperature so it doesn't get too warm. Such machines require diligently kept coldness. Patients, however, are allowed to lie shivering on an uncomfortable table covered only with a thin, minimally warm blanket. Apparently patients are expected to be more adaptable than machines.

After my scan and arriving back in my original room, I finally begin to warm up and calmly wait for the doctor to return with what I'm sure will be news of no significance. For the third time this afternoon, he appears from behind the blue curtain that blocks the doorway leading into the hall. This time his demeanor and body language look serious. He moves slowly, no longer smiles and appears concerned and unsure about what he should say. I realize all the talk about body language telling more than words is true.

"We found a mass in your left breast," he informs me. "It's about an inch in diameter."

I guess he doesn't want to waste any time. He says a few other things, but I have no idea what they are. The only words that matter are mass, breast and inch. Even the word "mass" sounds ominous, worrisome and overwhelmingly serious. You aren't supposed to have masses of anything in your body, are you?

I call my husband David because suddenly I am no longer feeling strong or invincible but rather can literally feel myself beginning to crumble. Minutes later he arrives, waits for me to get dressed and then listens to the doctor's grim words himself. Immediately I am scheduled for a diagnostic mammogram.

Maybe a heart attack would have been better.

-2-

First Appearance

Looking back, it's ironic that cancer made its grand entrance into my family's life on my birthday, as if trying to make some kind of ominous statement about life and death. I didn't know it at the time, but cancer was here to stay. February 1, 2004 was the date Mother discovered the tiny lump in her right breast, and cancer slithered into our lives for good. Such a thing is definitely not a milestone anyone wants to mark a birthday. My parents were planning a visit to my house that winter day to celebrate another birthday with daughter number three.

When I was a young girl, I asked my dad once if he was disappointed that cold February day when I was born to get the news he was once again the father of a baby girl. When I was born, fathers were forced to wait or pace around in waiting rooms while their wives labored in mysterious delivery rooms somewhere down the hall. Somehow fathers were considered to be unnecessary, unprepared or just inappropriate to directly participate in this life-changing event. Responding to my question, he laughed, shook his Elvis-like head of thick, black hair and of course said no, but I wondered how he could not have been a little disappointed for at least an instant back then. He must have wished for a son at least once or twice while waiting nine months for me to arrive. But there he was, a young father on a teacher's salary with three daughters ages four and under to feed, clothe and parent.

If he ever was disappointed, he never showed it. I could not have

7

had a better father. He was a hands-on dad before it was cool. I don't know how many diapers he changed, but he did "baby sit" us all the time, did a lot of the cooking, helped put us to bed, took us to doctor appointments, always bought the groceries and drove us wherever we needed to go. He had and still has more patience than any man I have ever known. I don't think I ever saw him really lose his temper. On one occasion he did threaten my sisters and me with a broken-off red stick of some sort when we had successfully maxed out his patience, but of course he never used it. And he was raised in a family where the rod was not spared.

When I was in high school, I had my dad for a history teacher. It was a small-town school, so there was no one else. At school he was a popular teacher. Kids liked him for his quirky mannerisms like looking at the clock every few seconds during lectures instead of at them and for his sense of humor, but mostly they knew he was fair and genuinely liked them. Having your father as your teacher could have been quite an awkward experience for a teenager, but luckily none of my friends thought much about it or gave me a hard time when I earned my A's from him. It felt good to have a father who knew so much about history, told jokes, stopped to talk to anyone he met in the grocery store, loved football and ran the scoreboard Friday nights. I was proud to be his daughter, even if I was number three.

On my 49th birthday, Mother called to cancel the birthday celebration. Canceling birthday celebrations, even for a daughter turning 49, was a serious matter. Mother loved birthdays and the marking off of each year as if it were another precious link she could add to her gold chain of motherhood, further increasing its value. On that birthday she called instead to tell me she had found a lump in her right breast and was going to the doctor the very next morning. As she delivered the news, she tried to sound calm and reassuring, but I immediately sensed the fear and uncertainty in her voice. Of course, I pretended to be calm as well and told her it would probably turn out to be nothing, thinking cancer couldn't possibly infiltrate into our lives. Cancer was a disease for other families, not ours.

After the initial appointment with her very competent, small-town doctor, it was determined she would go to the Twin Cities to have her biopsy. After all, I lived there at the time, and it seemed like the logical place to go for the best care. Mere days after my canceled birthday celebration, my parents, my brother Mark and one of my older sisters, Kay, and I filed into the Fairview Southdale Hospital Breast Center in Edina, Minnesota. Filled with apprehension as we walked through those doors, I contemplated how odd it was to have breast cancer so neatly compartmentalized. An entire facility devoted to breasts seemed to emphasize the seriousness of this disease and our predicament even further. That day was the beginning of our regimen of "going along to doctor appointments." The resulting biopsy report of that day proved Mother did indeed have breast cancer, making her another statistic to be tabulated, analyzed and thrown into the murky pool of cancer. I had stepped onto a bridge of sorts, connecting my old life where things felt safe and reliable, to my new, uncertain life, where my future no longer guaranteed me a mother. I didn't know it at the time, but cancer was in my life for good.

Many more appointments followed where we filled up stuffy waiting and exam rooms as if our strength in numbers would somehow give us more power over cancer. We became familiar with sitting on uncomfortable chairs specifically set aside for cancer patients and their families, where there was always bad coffee simmering nearby. Usually, there were also plates of chocolate chip, raisin and sugar cookies covered with clear plastic lids, as if coffee and cookies were at least two things to be counted on. Then there were the pamphlets, too many racks of pamphlets pretending to contain answers for cancer. There were pamphlets about what to expect from radiation or chemo, the importance of proper nutrition, where to find support groups and where to order hair pieces and wigs. I quickly realized the inadequacy of pamphlets. You can't sum up answers to cancer in tidy 4 x 8 pamphlets.

My mother felt tremendous guilt for bringing cancer into our family, a totally ridiculous way to feel. She was not even the first member of our extended family to get breast cancer. Both her sisters already had been diagnosed. But now cancer had permeated into the ring of our immediate family, and we could no longer feel sheltered and safe. Her guilt and anxiety seemed to grow daily. After all, mothers like to fix things, not be the source of unsolvable problems.

"I'm so sorry you'll have to think about this every year now on your birthday, Nancy," she repeated countless times, devastated that my birthday was forever tarnished and that she had been the one to tarnish it.

Despite being shaken up by the unexpected entrance of this intruder into our lives, we all started out optimistically, confidently believing if we just did things right, all would be well.

Isn't this how breast cancer is supposed to go? Follow the "how to do breast cancer handbook," and things will be fine. Isn't this the message most often delivered by The Pink Machine?

I was determined I would not be on that bridge for long. I was wrong.

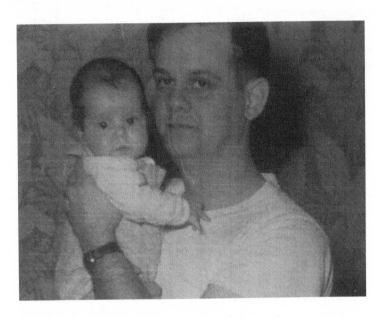

My dad and daughter #3—me!

-3-

Mammogram

Before I have my mammogram, I follow the technician into a small room to answer the same questions they asked me at my last mammogram. The room oozes pink. I know they planned it this way on purpose, but I'm thinking any color but pink would be better about now. In addition to two pink, cushiony chairs, the small room also has a desk and computer, various appropriately framed and hung technician certificates, soothing nature-type pictures and of course, a box of pink Kleenex. The technician's name is Nadine. She is young, caring and soft spoken.

Nadine begins to go through her standard list of questions, recording and compiling my personal data as if I am a person of worldly importance. At the end of her calculating, she hands me a piece of paper which states my risk of breast cancer to be 43.6 percent. This is before my mammogram. From the expression on her face, I can tell this is deemed to be pretty high, but I already know all the statistics. It's barely been two years since Mother died. Everything about breast cancer is still painfully familiar and clear in my mind.

The two of us head into the mammogram room, and she proceeds to take what feels like way too many pictures of my breasts. I stand, turn, hold my breath when asked and pretend I'm doing fine as my breasts are squeezed, squished, turned, angled and flattened into various shapes and positions they were never intended to be in. She takes extra shots of the left one, the one with secrets, the breast of betrayal.

Next, I am led into another room where I receive an ultrasound version done by a different technician, a second opinion, so to speak, by a second machine. I see the mass on the screen, and the technician clicks and records the dark, gray image unknown to me only a day ago. She continues to click, zoom, magnify and record. I hate that clicking sound.

I go back to the pink room to wait for results I already know. The mass is indeed confirmed. I have seen it with my own eyes. Still, the radiologist must deliver the news personally. The words must be said out loud. When he enters the tiny room a short time later, he shakes my hand, confirms the mass, briefly explains the next step (biopsy), asks me if I have any questions and then leaves, returning to his office down the hall where he studies pictures of other women's breasts.

Nadine returns. She is obviously well trained and quite compassionate; I think she actually has tears in her eyes, or maybe it's only that mine do.

-4-

The Letter, March 2006

For two years we managed to outmaneuver, or at least maneuver around Mother's cancer, quietly deceiving ourselves into believing we had successfully squelched it. Sometimes months went by and we didn't even talk about cancer, perhaps subconsciously thinking our silence would silence it as well. I was still standing on the bridge, but it felt stronger and more secure, leading me to believe I might be stepping off or turning around soon. Then the letter arrived, like a mysterious time bottle holding secrets about other lives somehow connected to ours, and once again my mother's life, and therefore mine as well, was thrown into more upheaval than even the day she was diagnosed. The letter was from Mother's biological sister's son. My family history is like a plot for some fiction novel or soap opera, but suddenly it was an important part of my new reality.

Years before, on my wedding day in fact, Mother somewhat hesitantly pulled me aside while we were casually making waffles to serve our relatives for brunch and proceeded to share a startling secret.

"Nancy, Grandma is not really my mother, so she isn't really your grandmother either," she said.

After a few moments of dead silence, I remember feeling irritated more than anything by the bizarrely timed announcement. I didn't want to think it could be true, or think about it at all really; it was my wedding day for crying out loud. Why would she want to tell me such a thing that day of all days? I was only 21 years old, and family skeletons seemed unimportant and irrelevant to me. *That revelation was the first unseen indicator about the future trajectory of my life some thirty years later.*

Despite the fact I wasn't interested in hearing such news, there was no stopping her. Mother was driven by some sense of urgency and went on to explain that her biological mother Julia had died shortly after Mother was born. No one knew for sure why Julia died. I have no idea what happened to Mother's father, my "real" grandfather, he was never mentioned. It was as if he never existed. Who knew there was so much mystery in my roots? Julia's sister, Clara (the grandmother I knew), had lost a baby daughter (Clarice) around the same time my mother was born. I remember walking through an old country church cemetery in North Dakota with my grandmother, mother and sisters one summer evening as a young girl looking at a grave with a simple marker for a baby Clarice. That was the only time she was ever mentioned, and I knew I wasn't supposed to ask questions even though I wanted to, so I didn't. For some reason my grandmother had chosen to never discuss Clarice, instead keeping the mystery hidden away in the unknown place deep within her heart where such secrets stayed buried. I still wonder about why Clarice died, the incredible pain Grandma endured those many years ago and why the ordeal was never discussed. Women back then thought it was too sad or just unacceptable to talk about such things. Now I think it's even sadder not to.

Clara and her husband Chester still desperately wanted a baby, so they willingly took in baby Jual and decided to raise her as their own. Such carefully guarded secrets had never before been revealed to me. I suppose my mother felt compelled to tell me this family history on my wedding day for whatever reason. So Mother was really my grandma's niece. My mother's two sisters were actually her cousins. These twists made no sense to me, and I put them out of my mind. What did it matter anyway? And it didn't, until many years later when the letter arrived.

The letter was about Muriel, my mother's biological sister, an aunt I never knew. How strange to suddenly have this unwelcome arm reaching out from the past, this sister and aunt who was really just a stranger. As far as I knew, my mother had never thought much about her real parents or other siblings she had out there. She had been raised in a loving and giving home. She had a family and needed no other. I have no idea when or how she had been told the truth about her other family.

Muriel had recently passed away, and her son was sending the letter. He had chosen to wait for his mother's death to make contact with my mother. I wondered if family discussions had been held in their house about this other family out there somewhere. Maybe Muriel had not wanted him to contact us. She had been living far away in Alaska, far removed from us even in the literal sense. Regardless, the ramifications of sending that letter were pretty great.

Within the letter was unsettling information. Muriel had led a difficult life, healthwise that is. She had developed breast cancer as well as ovarian and finally pancreatic. She died of the latter at the age of 82. The unsettling thing was the reason the letter had been sent. Muriel had completed genetic testing, and it was discovered she carried the BRCA2 gene mutation.

When functioning normally, the BRCA2 gene promotes healthy breast cell growth and repair. When it is mutated, it does not properly do its job. If a woman carries this BRCA2 gene mutation, it doesn't mean she will definitely get cancer, but her chances of developing breast cancer in her lifetime are significantly increased, as are her chances for ovarian and possibly pancreatic, colon, thyroid and melanoma cancers. [1]

After the letter arrived, Mother was a changed person. She felt tremendous guilt, even though obviously she had no control over the genes she long ago inherited. Likewise, no one had control over the genes my sisters, brother and I had inherited. She knew this, of course, but was still plagued with guilt and struggled over her decision to be tested or not. Of course, I always knew what her decision would be. We all did. I tried to be understanding, but I was not supportive. I did not want to know if she carried this mutated gene. If you go looking for answers, sometimes you find them, and I wasn't sure I wanted to. I wasn't ready yet.

"I made an appointment to have the test done," she called to inform me out of the blue on a September day. "Will you please go along with me? I need you to go along."

"Why would you schedule such an important appointment without discussing it with me first?" I asked.

---

[1] FORCE *(Facing Our Risk of Cancer Empowered) FacingOurRisk.org.* "Understanding BRCA & HBOC - Hereditary Cancers & Genetics."

I didn't even try to hide my annoyance with the whole situation. Why did she have to be so persistent? How could she lecture me now? I had my first mammogram at age 40. She did not have one until she found her lump. I tried not to sound upset, but I knew that was exactly how I did sound. I heard the hurt in her voice, and for some odd reason I was secretly glad about that.

Of course, I did agree to go along and made the two-hour drive from my home in Menomonie, Wisconsin, to the Mayo Clinic in Rochester, Minnesota. It was mid-October, and normally I would have admired the changing colors of the leaves on the trees covering the hills of the Mississippi River valley, but my mind was focused on more important things like blood tests, cancer and insistent mothers. The day was cloudy and gloomy, looking like rain, but that seemed appropriate for the appointment which seemed gloomy as well. I arrived in Rochester and followed the signs which all seemed to point to the city's focal point, Mayo Clinic. It is the epicenter of the entire city, almost a separate community itself. I parked in a ramp and met Mother, Dad, Kay and Mark somewhere beyond the main doors. We tried not to look overwhelmed by the hugeness and seriousness of the place, but I knew that was exactly how we did look. People with small health problems don't go to *the* Mayo Clinic.

Mayo has transformed sickness into a highly successful, organized business, so we didn't have to wait long. Soon Mother, Dad, Kay, Mark and I once again found ourselves sitting on folding chairs in a stuffy room not intended for so many people. A nurse asked us countless questions about our family history, and we tried to remember and answer most. She asked her questions methodically, gathering and recording every detail while completing intricate diagrams of our family tree as if she was solving some mysterious puzzle.

Next, a middle-aged, blond doctor specializing in genetics appeared and began to ask more questions, analyze our data and unlock secrets of our DNA. I could tell she did this all the time because she knew exactly what questions to ask and in what order to ask them. She looked so serious and brought out books with diagrams of genes and chromosomes, trying to make such matters easier for us to understand. I remembered tenth grade biology class when I studied such things long ago, but now as I looked at the geneticist's diagrams holding such serious information, all they did was remind me of ridiculous paper chains my friends and I used to make in junior high.

We collected and saved countless yellow Juicy Fruit and green Doublemint gum wrappers, folding and connecting them into long, worthless, origami-like paper chains whose only purpose was to be made longer. The drawings and configurations on the page we now stared at looked like those silly paper chains. My mind was playing serious tricks on me, and I couldn't concentrate properly.

"Are you willing to live with the information you find out if you decide to go ahead and get tested?" the blond doctor asked.

She spoke in such a serious voice, pretending she had no opinion on what our decision should be.

No, I muttered silently to myself. I didn't want to know such information, but of course Mother did. So we sat in another waiting room while they drew blood from her arm to uncover secrets I didn't want to know.

A few weeks later the results arrived, and they revealed Mother did indeed carry the dreaded mutation. There it was on official letterhead paper. They even put it in bold, dark print as if to further emphasize our doom. **Deleterious Mutation**. I thought it sounded more like some kind of mental illness. We weren't even surprised by the report; we expected bad news. We all now realized my sisters, brother and I also had a 50/50 chance of having this mutated gene. We were now a "tainted" lot.

Again, I felt Mother's guilt. She no longer worried for herself but rather for me and my siblings. She now had a new mission, convincing us to be tested as well. Suddenly she was obsessed with statistics, mammograms and dire predictions of cancer. Clearly she was irritated with daughters who did not want to talk about such things. She gave me articles about women choosing prophylactic mastectomies and oophorectomies, but worrying about something I didn't yet have felt wrong to me, and I didn't want to do it. I felt like a defiant and rebellious teenager refusing to listen to her mother, but at the same time I wondered if someday I would regret such decisions. Should I get rid of parts of my body before they turn against me? *Another omen I ignored.*

Even though I realized sharing this information was the right thing for him to do, I was still irritated with Muriel's son, a person I did not even know. What right did he have to suddenly cause all this worry and tension in my family? We were not his business or concern. We were not his family. But of course, genetically speaking, we were.

After some time, things finally quieted down, and Mother eventually quit nagging us about getting tested. She seemed to be doing quite well and continued having her follow-up oncology appointments. Maybe if we all kept quiet, cancer would too. Maybe I could still turn around on this damn bridge. Maybe things could get back to normal. Maybe we could stop thinking about cancer and mutated genes so much. Maybe we were done with cancer. Maybe...

-5-

Alone & Afraid, April 2010

Perhaps surprisingly, I spend the next few days feeling great, almost as if defying cancer, challenging it to show itself. I don't feel sick, therefore, I cannot *be* sick. I keep busy, getting things done I have been neglecting. Suddenly mundane, everyday chores don't seem that bad. I find walking around Target buying supplies and groceries is an outing worth enjoying. Doing laundry, cleaning scuzzy bathrooms and organizing my closets don't seem that bad either. Some kind of crazy nesting instinct has definitely kicked in.

This is the first time I have seriously thought about my own mortality. Now I have silly, crazy thoughts and questions, truly absurd ones like thoughts about me dying a slow, agonizing death, and will I be able to remain dignified through it all? Will it be painful? Who will be with me at my deathbed? Am I replaceable? Of course I am. How long will David wait until he starts dating again? Like I said, they were thoughts of the absurd kind.

I always just assumed David and I would grow old together. After all, we've been through a lot. We've been together some forty of my fifty-five years, which sounds amazing and impossible at the same time. Having someone in my life who loves and cares about me is a great gift and despite cancer, I feel lucky in this regard anyway. He takes care of telling the kids and reassures them things will be fine, even though neither one of us feels certain about this. I go shopping at the mall. I walk around soaking up the normalcy of it all—babies in strollers being pushed by busy moms, stores pretending to have sales, clerks looking unhappy with their jobs and racks of spring and summer clothing waiting to be tried on.

I'm having trouble sleeping at night. Usually I fall asleep fairly quickly but then wake up around 3 or 4 a.m., and my mind begins to overload itself with fearful thoughts about cancer, agonizing death and all the things I have not yet accomplished in my life. I begin making mental notes about what I will write in the next chapter of my book, or maybe I will need to write a whole new book, the one that I write about dying. I tell myself how silly I am for having such thoughts, but the sensible, reasonable part of my brain feels weak and overpowered in the middle of the night.

I've already decided I am very different from Mother in two ways. First of all, I don't like a lot of people coming along to doctor appointments. She loved it when we filled up waiting rooms or hovered around waiting for nurses, doctors or test results. Not me. The fewer people hovering the better. This is not really surprising, me being more of an introvert. Mother was not an introvert. Secondly, I don't mind the waiting. Mother did. I like the waiting. The way I figure it, bad news will find me soon enough. I enjoy each day with no bad news, or no news at all. I am in no hurry.

I read a quote today that went something like, "You are never really all alone in anything, but you are all alone in almost everything." It makes perfect sense. I know I am not alone, but yet I feel totally alone. I also feel afraid, the two A-words, alone and afraid.

Today David and I meet with a surgeon. His name is Dr. Ross. I think it's odd to meet with a surgeon when no surgery is planned yet, but again there is that protocol to follow. For some reason Dr. Ross has a calming air to him immediately when he enters the room. He looks like a doctor who knows what he is doing, although I'm not sure why. Fair or not, some of Mother's doctors did not. They did not exude confidence. Dr. Ross is tall and bald. Maybe the baldness thing is a unique, immediate source of comfort for patients staring cancer in the face. Who knows? Again, he asks for details about my symptoms and dates for things like when I started menstruating, and on the other end of the female reproductive spectrum, when I hit menopause. He was surprised and chuckled when I pinpointed my exact age and grade when I had my first period. I was eleven.

Men have it easy, or at least easier. They don't have dates or memories like that to carry around. I will not forget the day of my first period. I hated the "arrival of womanhood." Mostly I hated those bulky pads that were uncomfortable, leaky and downright disgusting. Luckily, they had "prepared" the girls somewhat in school by showing us a movie about our changing bodies and what to expect, even though after watching it, we still had no idea. The boys were not allowed to see this movie but were instead told the girls were watching a movie on babysitting. Even back then, the idea of such secrecy seemed ludicrous to me.

You won't have another period for quite a while after your first one, Mother had mentioned a few times, sounding like she knew what she was talking about, so I believed her.

She was wrong. A month or so later, I was sitting at my desk, excused myself and was horrified in the restroom to find out I was already having another one. There were not even any tampon or pad dispensers hanging on the wall, so I just left. I mean what was a girl to do? I guess girls in elementary school weren't supposed to have periods yet. So I simply left the building and walked home telling no one (especially my male teacher). When I walked through the back door, Mother was washing dishes. Seeing me at that time of day was a surprise of course.

"What in the world are you doing home?" she asked.

"You were *wrong*, it came again already," I said.

Immediately I headed for the privacy of our bathroom; such things are not easily forgotten.

Dr. Ross asks me if I can feel the lump, and I tell him I was finally able to find it this morning while in the shower. I feel embarrassed to have so much trouble zeroing in on my cancer's location within my own body. He does an exam with his nurse hovering, and immediately I like her. She looks kind and experienced with her gray hair and wrinkles. Her concern feels genuine. Her name is Jenny.

"I think your lump is free-floating and not attached to your chest wall," Dr. Ross says.

This is good news, but I don't know why.

"I don't feel anything in your lymph nodes either."

More good news. We all know cells are microscopic, so this isn't really good news of much value, but it's a glimmer and we'll take it. We take glimmers of good news now. David waits and listens on the other side of the curtain as if he has never seen my breasts before.

Cancer protocol is so weird.

Finally my exam is over and I am allowed to get dressed. The three of us talk in a huddled conference.

"Your mass is rated a 5 on a scale of 1 to 5," Dr. Ross says. "This is due to the size of it and your family history. It's a *concern*."

There's that word mass again, a despicable word, plus the fresh reminder about my tainted gene pool. And a new word, concern. My mass is a concern, a double whammy. We spend the next twenty minutes or so asking questions, some with answers but many without. The nurse leaves to get going on scheduling my now deemed urgent biopsy. We all shake hands, and David and I leave the office feeling vulnerable yet confident. We are taking action. My biopsy will be Tuesday. It's Friday. Nurse Jenny succeeds at getting me in quickly, and I wonder if my file has the word "urgent" stamped on it.

After we leave the clinic, David pulls into the Culver's parking lot so we can get dinner, just as we had planned. He parks the car, and for the first time I am irritated with him.

"How can you possibly be hungry?" I ask.

I cannot open the door, but instead start crying as I sit frozen, holding the door handle.

"Go through the drive-through," I order him and not very nicely, not nicely at all.

When we get home, we sit on the sofa and I continue crying, making loud, obnoxious, sobbing and snorting noises. I sound disgusting, even to myself. I am angry, no, I am fuming. Why is this happening to me? David tries to hold and comfort me, but I am unholdable. I am not able to be comforted either. He doesn't know what to say or do; who would?

Finally, I allow my hungry husband to get off the sofa to go eat his cold chicken dinner.

-6-

Unwelcome News, September 2007

"I want to go back to the North Shore one more time soon," Mother announced.

She made this announcement in August at the end of a hurried visit I had made to my parents' house. It was such a seemingly innocent proclamation that went unnoticed.

The North Shore of Lake Superior is a beautiful destination. The scenery in the area rivals any other, and more people are discovering its majestic forests, lookout bluffs, rocky shorelines and pebbly beaches every year. It is a place of remarkable, pristine serenity no matter what time of year you visit. Each season displays its own unique version of beauty almost as if trying to outdo the others.

On a clear day in summer, the lake is breathtakingly blue and seems to continue on forever into the horizon looking more like an ocean than a lake, and you immediately understand why it bears the name Superior. Often you can observe ships with their loads of iron ore or grain. From a distance the huge vessels look like bathtub toys moving over the water as they follow their familiar routes through the Great Lakes and the St. Lawrence Seaway, ending up many miles to the east. Summer brings numerous tourists and camping enthusiasts to the well-known destinations like Split Rock Lighthouse, which boldly juts out on a bluff as if begging to be noticed, and Gooseberry Falls, where the unexpected sights and sounds of cascading water take visitors by surprise. In summer these places seem crowded and noisy, overflowing with parents unsuccessfully attempting to keep their children close by.

Fall on the North Shore is spectacular if you hit the color change just right and even if you don't. Leaves turning golden with vast blue expansions of sky and water for the backdrop are sights people now drive many miles to see. The locals complain over their coffee about all the Twin Cities invaders, but yet these are the very people responsible for pumping much needed dollars into their businesses and wallets.

Winter is perhaps most stunning. Maple and birch trees intertwined with pines seem to stand taller and straighter as if defying the elements, saying, we can survive until spring. The trunks of the birch trees are now unobstructed by leaves and boldly show off the stark whiteness of their bark. The lake begins to form ice along its shores, and the snow starts accumulating, waiting for noisy skiers to arrive.

Early spring is my favorite time to visit the North Shore. This is mostly because it's the quietest time; there aren't as many visitors. Despite the calendar it's really still winter, but there's a feeling it might soon be over. The snow and ice formations on the rocky shores are spectacular and starting to break up. There is no other sound or sight quite like crashing waves thundering over a still-frozen shoreline that is trying to unthaw but somehow knows it is not quite time. The best place to marvel at such things is at a favorite resort relaxing in front of an expansive window next to a roaring fire. If you visit those popular tourist places now, they are empty, quiet, peaceful and somehow more spectacular, giving you the feeling they are there just for your enjoyment. Segments of the waterfalls are still frozen into ghostly icicle configurations, and the campgrounds and visitor centers are almost empty.

The North Shore is also special because many facilities still allow you the privilege of bringing your dog, and dogs, too, seem to love this place. We have taken many of our dogs to the North Shore over the years. Nothing compares with standing on treacherous, rocky shores or hiking on a still snow-covered trail in early spring while accompanied by your dog who laps up the sights, sounds and smells. At the end of the day when you both unwind in front of a warm fire, you know the bond you share has deepened even further.

Mother loved the North Shore, and it was always one of her favorite travel destinations. That September trip turned out to be her last. In fact, it was her last September, period. While she was there, she experienced new and unaccounted for pain in her shoulder. Even though she didn't tell us right away, she was growing suspicious.

Shortly after that trip it was time for a checkup, scans and a meeting with her oncologist, who gave us the news no cancer patient ever wants to hear, the news of recurrence.

"Your mother's scan shows spots on her ribs and possibly on her spine," he said.

Did he think calling cancer cells "spots" was a gentler way to give bad news?

"We will need to schedule more tests to take a closer look."

I wondered what mysterious force caused cancer cells deep within her body to suddenly reawaken. Did we too easily forget about them? It seemed we were in some sort of "chess match" with cancer as our opponent, and we were strategically maneuvering our pieces around the board trying to protect our queen. Had we not pondered our moves carefully enough?

I was forced to step back onto the bridge I never wanted to be on.

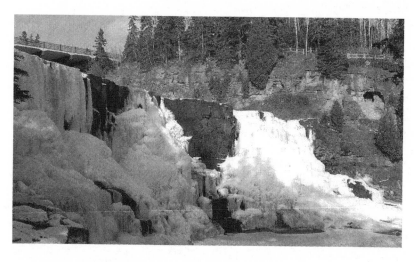

Gooseberry Falls in November 2014. Beautiful & spectacular even when frozen. The North Shore was one of my mother's favorite destinations. It's one of mine too.

-7-

Biopsy

Today, April 27, is my biopsy day. This day brings us a step closer to getting answers I'm not sure I want. David and I drive to the hospital in Eau Claire, Wisconsin. He reaches over to hold my hand, mostly driving with his other free hand the entire trip. I wonder if he is as frightened as me. I've read about the biopsy procedure I will be having, core needle biopsy. I was with Mother when she had hers. I know what to expect, yet I do not have a clue.

The HERS Breast Center, part of the local hospital, is set up to be as nonthreatening and relaxing as possible, but it's almost like they're trying too hard. Still, knowing compassion is mixed in with the decor and surroundings does make a difference. Sort of. There are padded chairs in the waiting room, soft music plays, coffee simmers, books are available to read, pink (too much of it) is everywhere, stain-glass artwork hangs in the windows where sunlight streams in and there is a general feel in the air of femininity, respect, caring and empathy but not pity. I am grateful for this as I'm sure every woman who walks through the door is as well.

Another woman is waiting too. She looks considerably older than me, and I feel resentful, even a little angry, that I am here doing this already. I am even envious of Mother. She didn't have to deal with any of this shit until she was 74, and here I am two decades younger facing this crap. I know such thoughts are ridiculous; it's not like there is a good age to get cancer. There isn't. I don't get to stay angry for very long; I'm too scared, and today fear trumps anger. Another man sits waiting for his wife, and he looks older too. David sits down, and I pace, but not for long. A nurse or technician comes right away to take me back. Her name is Kris. She doesn't wear a uniform, just regular clothes, another attempt at normalcy. She looks young and is very friendly. I like her instantly.

The changing area has dim lights and dark, wooden cabinetry that feels somehow warm and comforting. After changing into my pink, flowered gown, Kris escorts me to the procedure room where I lie on a narrow table that feels like I will roll off if I turn, move at all or even blink an eye. Kris covers me with a warm blanket which immediately makes me more relaxed. I am starting to love warmed-up blankets. We make conversation, and I look around the dimly lit room which again is discreetly appointed with soothing pictures of flowers, seashells and other nature stuff.

Momentarily, my new radiologist, Dr. Vincent, enters the room, and I notice she has large breasts except hers, of course, are cancer free. I listen carefully as she explains the procedure, and I wonder how many biopsies she does in a day's work. She describes, and I listen and nod as if it's all no big deal.

"Do you have any questions?" she asks, but I understand too much for my own good.

"No," I say. "Let's just get it over with."

I watch the entire procedure on a computer screen. I see the monster, the mass, there in plain sight looking shadowy and evil as if able to plot against me. The tiny mass is only a clump of cells but right now totally controls what will happen to my life next.

The needle stings a bit as it delivers the local anesthetic which immediately takes effect, thank God. It doesn't feel much different than a shot of Novocain at the dentist. Next, the big-breasted doctor pushes on my much-smaller-than-hers breast and wiggles the needle in there, guided by the ultra-sound image that I pray is accurate.

"I'm going to take the first sample now," Dr. Vincent says, preparing me for the first jolt.

Immediately there is a popping sound, sort of like a nail or staple gun. That's when the sample is cut, sucked up and collected. It sounds worse than it is. She takes five more samples, and each time I jump even though I know what's coming. Each zap is a startling, unexpected jolt that makes me jump, and I wonder what might happen if I were to roll off the narrow table. What if no one caught me?

"Be sure you get enough," I say. "I don't want to come back."

I have heard stories about women having to come back.

"Oh, I am," she reassures me. "They probably only need one or two samples, and we are taking six, each the size of a grain of rice."

Within ten minutes it's all over, and Kris is applying pressure. After a few more minutes, another nurse comes in to relieve Kris, who takes my samples of mysterious information to the lab. Once again I wonder if mine is a rush order. Katie, the new nurse, is cheerful and talkative. We talk about dogs, breasts and how to take care of my new little incision.

"You look fabulous," she tells me as she helps me off the table.

How can you not love someone who tells you this when you know it isn't true?

I get dressed, and they send me on my way with my little gel ice pack, directions on what to do at home and promises to keep me in their thoughts. David looks surprised to see me appear from behind closed doors so soon. I feel relieved and temporarily happy. We both do. We have survived another step. It wasn't even that horribly bad.

I spend much of the rest of the day stretched out on our blue, leather sofa in the family room applying ice packs every hour for fifteen minutes at a time. David waits on me, reassures me, but mostly just loves me. We watch Rambo movies on AMC. I have never seen a Rambo movie. Mindless TV viewing is exactly what I need about now.

Links to the Past, October 2007

Madelia is a small, rural community in southern Minnesota with a population of about 2,500 and was the only home I knew growing up. It is one of those typical small-town communities full of hidden history, much like hundreds of others across the Midwest, one more small town just trying to survive.

The people of Madelia like to boast that the notorious Younger brothers Bob, Cole and Jim, along with Charlie Pitts, were captured outside of town. In September 1876, the Younger brothers, along with Pitts, Jesse and Frank James, as well as a couple other lesser-known outlaws, had attempted to rob the bank in Northfield, Minnesota, about 100 miles to the northeast. Plans of their intended robbery had leaked out, quickly unraveled and resulted in a bloody shootout on the streets of Northfield. The Younger brothers, Frank and Jesse James and Pitts, all wounded, headed south to escape the manhunt. Posses were set up throughout the region, and the manhunt continued for days. A local posse was rounded up in Madelia as well. The Madelia posse succeeded in capturing the Younger brothers and mortally wounding Pitts on September 21, 1876. Frank and Jesse James managed to escape, heading on to Missouri. But the villainous James-Younger Gang was no more.[2] Madelians are still quite proud

---

[2] *Wikipedia.* "James-Younger Gang. Northfield, Minnesota Raid."

of their town's legendary accomplishment, and the locals sometimes reenact the event in September.

Like many small towns, Madelia was a great place to grow up, but most of my classmates had no intention of staying and neither did I. After high school graduation, the majority of us ended up leaving for college or employment opportunities elsewhere. I left too.

Many residents of such small towns understandably harbor resentment toward those larger neighboring cities that end up enticing away their young people, slowly chipping away at their town's future. Growing up I often heard talk about Twin Citians as if they were foreigners from a faraway country, not fellow residents of the same state a mere 100 miles to the north.

In Madelia and the surrounding areas, people shortened the name Twin Cities down even further to just "the cities." When you talked about going to or coming from Minneapolis or St. Paul, they were always referred to as "the cities." I always wondered how far out that radius of understanding extended. How far would I have to travel to reach a destination where the inhabitants would no longer know exactly where I was talking about when I mentioned "the cities"?

Even though we lived only about 100 miles south of the cities, our trips there were few and far between when I was growing up. The rare trips we did take were carefully planned and something to look forward to with almost a vacation-like feel. Once a year or so, we made the trek just to shop at Southdale Center in Edina, a Minneapolis suburb. Southdale, with its three levels of seemingly endless stores, was the mega mall of that time long before the Mall of America put the neighboring suburb of Bloomington on the map. A handful of times we ventured even further on into St. Paul and visited Como Park Zoo for the day. The zoo was free, and after we finished wandering around there looking at animals in cages, we spent a few more hours at the adjacent amusement park going on rides until we ran out of tickets and money.

Dad was always relieved to put that city traffic behind him, get back on U.S. Highway 169 South and finally Highway 60, the two-lane highway that led us back home to Madelia. Mother couldn't help with the driving since she never did obtain her license, something that seemed unfathomable to her children, but worked out fine for my parents. I remember a few occasions when Dad handed over the wheel to her, and she would nervously practice driving on quiet country roads with a spellbound, captive audience in the backseat, but she never did pursue that piece of plastic. I don't need a license, she often proclaimed, and she really didn't because Dad patiently drove her wherever she wanted to go, or else she walked.

Eventually, even Highway 60 became four lanes, and suddenly Madelia had more than one exit you could choose from to enter our town. Unfortunately, that also meant drivers didn't need to exit at all and could just keep on going.

After David and I graduated from college and got married, we looked forward to escaping small-town life and living anonymously in the Twin Cities. But once I got there and even after I lived there for years, I never quite felt like I fit in there either. I was uncertain where my loyalty should be. I still felt like a small-town girl. Yet when I returned to Madelia, I was now from the cities and one of "those people." I didn't belong in either place.

My dad's birthday is October 3, so when the day arrived, I traveled to Madelia like usual to celebrate and check on Mother. Despite illness, birthday celebrations must continue. I couldn't show up empty handed, so I stopped along the way to buy a marble birthday cake decorated with too much gaudy, fall-colored frosting.

After dinner and birthday cake, Mother, Dad, Kay, Mark and I sat around in the living room trying to continue Dad's birthday celebration as if that year was no different than any other. We were all thinking about those darn mysterious spots. Observing Mother, I could tell she had a strong inclination as to the seriousness of the latest news, some kind of intuition only she had about her body. Mark was sitting on the floor in front of the glowing gas fireplace holding Radar, his black cairn terrier, when he finally broke the silence.

"The doctor didn't actually say the spots were cancer," he said.

"He sure did," Mother said.

As she spoke, she stiffened and sat upright in her chair as if positioning herself for heated debate. She seemed to be defending the seriousness of her situation, perhaps preparing us for something she already knew.

"You are in denial," I said. "You should try to be more sensitive to how Mother is feeling. This is her disease and these are her feelings, regardless of what your opinions are."

"Well, no one really wants to hear what I have to say anyway," he said.

"This is not about you, it's about Mother."

The more I spoke, the more friction I created. Why couldn't I just shut up?

Mark shook his head, and we continued to irritate each other while Mother, Dad and Kay sat there listening, saying little, until Mother finally ended up in tears. I felt badly about that, but I couldn't sit there and keep quiet. I wanted to scream, not be quiet. Quietness made me feel more upset and even more helpless.

"My cancer is just like Elizabeth Edwards'," Mother said.

She stated this with conviction, pleased to have some sort of breast cancer badge of allegiance with such a person.

What? And no, I thought to myself. You are twenty years older than Elizabeth Edwards, so you are not really alike. But, of course, I kept quiet. I could not strip her of her badge. That would have been too cruel.

Later that month after more appointments, more tests and more consultations, Mother's recurrence was confirmed, and she started on what we hoped would be our next wonder drug.

"Cancer grows really slowly in the bones, and this drug will slow it down even more," her oncologist said.

He sounded quite certain, so we believed him.

We remained optimistic, telling ourselves we were lucky to have discovered the spots so early. After all, if diagnosing breast cancer early initially is a good thing, shouldn't diagnosing a recurrence early on be a good thing too? I still had lots to learn about this damn disease and did not yet fully grasp the seriousness of our new situation.

A few days later, David and I planned a fall getaway and left for a weekend to look at fall color, but really we were escaping from responsibility and cancer. We drove on quiet backroads that wound and meandered to Galena, Illinois, the historic town famous for being the home of President Grant. Darkness arrived suddenly because it was now mid-October, and when we arrived in town, we strained our eyes looking for street signs to direct us.

We finally arrived at the doorstep of The Victorian Mansion, one of many Victorian-style bed and breakfasts in town. Perfectly positioned on top of a hillside, it seemed luxurious and extravagant, far removed from waiting and exam rooms where you couldn't breathe. It had a large foyer, a formal dining room and a parlor where all you were supposed to do was sit and relax on cushiony sofas and chairs that had velvety upholstery unlike the uncomfortable, unpadded folding chairs hastily set up in exam rooms. The whole mansion glistened with white-colored lights inside and out, and even in that place I was reminded of Mother. She loved white lights and always wanted a Victorian doll house. We even gave her one once for her birthday but never succeeded in getting it put together.

Our Galena Victorian Mansion had rooms on three floors, and ours was on the top with a spectacular view of the town that also glowed with the warmth of gentle white lights. The room had recently been remodeled with modern amenities added like a hot tub, a new shower and plush robes because visitors now days require modern conveniences while enjoying old-fashioned charm. When you entered that place, time seemed to know about slowing down, and the only expectations were about rest, privacy and solitude.

Saturday brought with it a perfect, unexpectedly warm autumn day. After a good night's rest and being served a delicious hot breakfast of quiche, fruit and hot coffee, we almost forgot about hospitals and cancer. Almost. We walked out onto the front porch decorated with pumpkins and a wooden witch and breathed in the clear, crisp air that didn't smell like a clinic or sickness. A gray cat with straggly fur strolled slowly around the porch, stopping periodically to lick its paws and stare at us, as if suggesting we shouldn't be there.

At day's end, after a hodge-podge of relaxing, walking and shopping, David and I found ourselves again on the front porch sitting in rocking chairs probably looking like some old couple. I gazed down at the town below while sipping wine and nibbling on cheese and crackers. We exchanged pleasantries and made small talk with a heavy-set pharmacist and his wife from Chicago.

Even there on that porch, my thoughts tumbled back to Mother and the almost unbearably hot August of 2001 when Kay, Mother, my daughter Lindsay and niece, Rachel, also made a trip to Galena. It was one of those girls-only trips, full of shopping, eating chocolate, touring Grant's home, endless talking and giggling and little sleep. Back then, we walked around town innocently, still unaware of cancer's intrusive ugliness yet to invade our lives.

Such memories, though sad and nostalgic, also made me feel at peace and grateful. I realized how intricately woven my mother was into every part of my life, even on a fall getaway to Galena, Illinois.

I also realized I would not be getting off that bridge anytime soon.

-9-

There Is "a" Cancer There

Today is April 29, just another ordinary spring day for most. For me, it is the day I wait for the biopsy result which will determine my future. So much is riding on one little phone call. I keep busy all morning long, confident no news will be delivered early in the day. Doctors make such phone calls at the end of their work days, I tell myself. I busy myself with more cleaning, more laundry and more journaling, but mostly more waiting. As the day goes by, I start feeling more and more on edge. It must be bad news. Bad news will be delivered late in the day. It will be put off because who wants to deliver bad news?

For much of the afternoon, I stretch out on the sofa and attempt to settle in with my latest Grisham novel, but I only pretend to concentrate. The only storyline I can concentrate on is my own. Elsie, our golden retriever, and Sophie, our English springer spaniel, wait with me. I decide to give the clinic until 4 p.m. to call, and then I will call them. Minutes tick away on the large, round clock behind the TV, but no call comes; 4 p.m. comes and goes too. I wait another ten minutes. Those minutes pass as well, and I determine I'll wait just five more.

Finally, I realize I cannot wait any longer or everyone at the clinic will be leaving for the day, and I will be forgotten. I muster up enough courage, make the call and leave a message with the receptionist who promises to deliver it to my doctor right away.

Minutes later, my doctor's nurse calls and says, "Nancy, your doctor isn't in this afternoon. I don't have your results. I am so sorry."

"What? Well, I'm sorry, too, but this is totally unacceptable," I say.

Immediately my heart starts racing and anger starts to rise up, but I know I cannot let it burst out. You cannot allow yourself to become too angry with people who are supposed to be on your side. Plus, it's not the nurse's fault. I take a deep breath to calm myself.

"I have an oncology appointment already scheduled for tomorrow morning at 9 a.m. You cannot expect me to walk into that appointment without first knowing my results," I say.

"Oh, I know. You're absolutely right," the nurse says. "I'll see what I can do."

Immediately I feel calmer and confident she will come through with some information. Nurses like her exude confidence. Nurses like her understand. I go back to the sofa but cannot sit still. I begin to pace around the room.

About thirty minutes later, my cell phone rings. I am afraid to answer it, and for an instant I think about pretending I am not available. If I don't answer, I cannot receive bad news today. I take another deep breath, grab my pen and paper and decide to answer. I might as well get it over with. After identifying himself and making sure he is speaking with the right person, this unknown-to-me doctor delivers the words I somehow knew were coming, but am still unprepared to hear.

"Well, there is a cancer there, your biopsy tested positive," he says.

His voice sounds too calm, too detached and too familiar with giving such news. I wonder why he calls it "a" cancer, not just cancer, like it really matters.

"What else can you tell me?" I ask.

What a ridiculous question. At this moment, what else matters?

"Well, that's all this report tells us really."

"I don't believe that," I snap back. "There has to be more."

He irritates me. I know he is doing me a favor, delivering this news to a patient who isn't even his. He didn't have to do this. He could have made me wait.

"There must be something more you can tell me," I say.

For some reason I don't trust him and feel as if he is not telling me everything, although I have no idea what he might be leaving out.

"The only other thing," he concedes, "is it says here you are grade one."

"Well, that's at least a bit of good news."

I know I probably sound more than a bit desperate.

"No, not really, it's the least important piece of information when we stage cancer," he says. "Tumor size, biology and number of lymph nodes involved are far more important pieces to the puzzle than grade."

My displeasure with this guy grows, even though I know he's right. I also know I am being unfair and judgmental, but I want to scream at him, what is your problem? Instead I keep pressing him for something further. I'm not sure what.

After I have squeezed all the information I will get out of him, I apologize for putting him on the spot and being so short. However, I don't really believe he deserves an apology, and I wonder if he knows I am insincere. I don't give a crap. As our conversation concludes, I start to tremble, and my voice beings to waver.

"Are you okay?" he asks, hearing me start to cry.

No, you asshole! You just told me I have cancer! These are the words with which I want to lash out, but of course this is impossible. Even he seems to suddenly realize his last remark sounded insensitive because his voice immediately softens.

"I know you've just been told you have cancer, and it's understandable for you to be upset," he says.

His concern and compassion come too late. I'm done with him.

We say our goodbyes and hang up. He probably goes home to have a nice quiet dinner with his wife and kids thinking no more about cancer today. I, on the other hand, start sobbing as I absorb the reality of my new life, for it feels my old life is over. Now I have cancer and am forever changed. I feel alone, angry, terrified, cheated, guilty, jinxed, unfairly treated and just plain miserable. I hear myself weeping and feel my body rocking back and forth, but it seems as if I am observing someone else's life, a person I do not recognize.

I am alone but not totally. Elsie and Sophie sit next to me and wonder what is wrong. Sophie puts her front paws up on the sofa and tries to lick my face. Elsie sits as close to me as she can get, wiggling her body as she tries to nudge Sophie out of the way. They somehow sense the seriousness of the situation. My dogs are the only ones to witness firsthand my ugliest moments. They are familiar with this role, consoling me only months earlier when I grieved for Mother who died from, of all things, breast cancer. Will I die from it too? Perhaps being alone with my dogs is for the best; they will never reveal the secrets they witness on a late afternoon in spring.

Finally, the voice deep within me that decides enough tears have flowed for now, summons me to stop, and I pull myself together. I collapse on the sofa, worn out and ashamed for crying more today than on the day Mother died. On top of everything else, I must be shallow and self-centered. I am a bad daughter too.

About thirty minutes pass and I hear the backdoor open. Poor David enters the house, reluctantly I'm sure, unaware of what he must deal with tonight. Elsie and Sophie immediately run to greet him, and he knows his answer because I do not follow. I wonder if he wishes he could turn around and leave. I would like to.

He wisely takes his time changing clothes, allowing me a few more minutes to be alone. I mindlessly turn on *ABC World News Tonight with Diane Sawyer,* and I am envious of her cancer-free life. Ironically, one of the news stories is about some sort of possible cancer vaccine, one for prostate cancer, not breast cancer. It's a potentially major breakthrough, perhaps to be available in five years.

"Wouldn't you know it, naturally the breakthrough will come for a man's cancer first," I say out loud to no one.

David comes into the family room, slowly sits down beside me and gently puts his arms around me. He says nothing; there is no need. It's been confirmed for him too. He is now a man with a wife who has "a" cancer. His old life is over too.

We don't get to sit around feeling sorry for ourselves very long. Cancer doesn't allow for that. In the morning we have our first appointment with Dr. Nambudiri, my oncologist. It seems impossible I need such a person in my life.

After a night of little sleep, I'm not sure I will be able to hold myself together at our appointment, but miraculously somehow I do. I must. I have to pay attention. The nurse who checks us in is named Joan. She is almost annoyingly nice, and then I realize she is an oncology nurse. She deals with cancer patients, even dying patients. She has to be nice; it's part of her job description. She realizes I'm a fresh one, newly diagnosed. "Cancer Newbie" might as well be stamped onto my forehead.

Waiting in the exam room feels like deja vu. Just like Mother. It's happening again. Just like Mother. Only this time it's *me*. Like usual, the room is tiny and poorly ventilated. Unfriendly fluorescent lighting glares and buzzes. Sitting on my chair, I fidget nervously because it seems if I sit too still I will more easily crumble.

When Dr. Nambudiri finally appears, we are openly relieved. After studying him briefly, as well as his certificates hanging on the wall, it is obvious he is from a different corner of the world, and I wonder how he ended up in Wisconsin. All I want is for him to be competent and knowledgeable. Compassionate would be a nice bonus. Almost immediately we realize he is all of these things and more. His demeanor is calm and serious as he listens to my now familiar story about how I ended up here. He listens attentively, asks questions about family history and carefully writes down my answers as if I am giving him important pieces to a puzzle, which I guess I am. I am the puzzle. Next he listens to me breathe and examines my lymph glands.

"I don't feel anything evident in your lymph glands so your cancer probably hasn't spread," he says.

Hearing him call it "your cancer" sounds odd because I realize this cancer does indeed belong to me. Such ownership feels unimaginable. I don't want to own my cancer.

"I don't think your chest pain is related. I think you did injure yourself raking, and it's unrelated to your cancer," he adds.

He sounds like he knows what he's talking about, so we believe him.

"Don't I need a chest x-ray or scan of some kind?" I ask.

How much proof do I need anyway?

"You had the CT scan in the ER, a mammogram, an ultrasound and your biopsy," he says. "Nothing else was picked up."

These are the best words I hear today.

At the conclusion of our appointment, we all concur it is essential for me to have the blood test to determine if I carry the BRCA2 gene mutation like Mother. If I have the mutated gene, a bilateral mastectomy will most certainly be recommended. If I do not have the gene mutation, there may be other options. I don't like any of the options. It's a joke to call them options. These are not options. You can turn down options. Actually, I guess I could turn these down, but then… well, the dying option sucks.

Surprisingly, I'm still fairly calm. I guess I am in cancer shock or something. I no longer fear the words bilateral mastectomy so much.

What I fear are words like stage IV, untreatable, unclear lymph nodes and chemotherapy. And oh yes, dying.

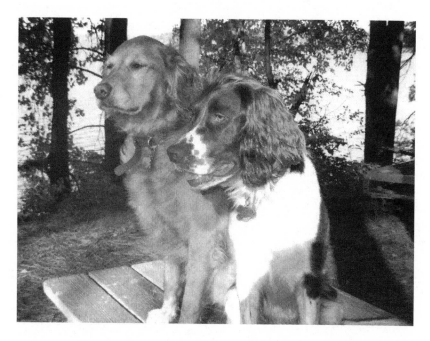

Elsie & Sophie, my special eyewitnesses & secret keepers

-10-

Decline

November brought chillier days and still more decline in Mother's health. I arrived in Madelia again to attend a bridal shower for my nephew's fiancée.

"I might just skip the shower," Mother said.

Clearly she thought it was too much effort to go, and she was probably right.

"It might make you feel better to get out," I said.

I hoped I sounded convincing rather than annoying.

Finally she gave in, got dressed up in her black pants and flowered, fall-colored, corduroy blazer, put on her red lipstick and reluctantly went with me. We sat at a long table in the basement of Kay's church eating quiche and fruit while she complained that the servings were too big. We visited with family and friends, managing to have a fairly good time.

A few acquaintances mentioned Mother's yellow appearance. Why would anyone bring up such a thing? I was immediately returned to the real world of cancer. I don't think Mother heard, or at least she pretended not to notice. The shower couldn't end fast enough for both of us.

Back at my parents' house I stretched out on the bed I used to sleep on as a girl and studied the bulletin board which still hung on the blue wall and was still covered with a mish-mash of photos, dried up flowers, newspaper clippings and various mementos my mother had never taken down. I looked at the faces of my siblings and I, all of us looking young and innocent, stuck there on that bulletin board where time could not reach us.

After reminiscing for a while, I called Susan, my oldest sister, and gave her a report on the shower and Mother's mood. Susan is four years older than me and has lived in Tennessee for years. She and her oldest son Michael were planning to come in a week or so. Susan was sensing the urgency we all felt and had decided not to delay her visit any longer.

"Just knowing you two are coming will give Mother something to look forward to and make her feel better," I said.

I was confident a visit from her first-born daughter and first-born grandchild would make a world of difference.

I have always been a little envious of Susan's elite, first-born status. Birth order is an intriguing topic. Being number three out of four puts you in an awkward position. You are not the first born with all that special, undivided attention. You are not the tail-ender or baby of the family. You are not even really in that precarious position of middle child, sort of, but not really. They say much is expected from first-born children; they are often overachievers. The baby is often considered to be the most loved, overly loved or just plain spoiled. The middle child is sometimes said to be left out, overlooked or kind of lost in the shuffle. But where does being three out of four put you? Stuck in the middle somewhere I guess.

Actually, that's exactly where I invariably did end up when my family traveled anywhere in the car when I was growing up. My spot was always in the middle of the backseat between Kay and Susan. I complained about the unfairness of that arrangement, of course, but to no avail. The pecking order was well established and quite permanent. I rarely sat elsewhere.

That seating arrangement wasn't so bad on short trips, but on the long family road trips we often took in the summer, I really felt the injustice of my position. Every summer, we made the 400-mile trip from Madelia to Park River, North Dakota, to visit my grandparents, and some summers we traveled to the West Coast passing through various national parks. On all of those trips, Susan and Kay had the luxury of each having her own window to look out and actually see the sights of wherever it was we happened to be traveling. Also, having a place to rest your head was something I was pretty envious of.

Those trips were all made long before mini-vans with third-row seating and DVD players, and if there were air-conditioned vehicles available then, we did not have one.

Of course, Mark also sat in the middle, but since he was the youngest and smallest, he always sat in the front seat between my parents. Somehow even that position seemed better than that of daughter number three, stuck in the middle.

Susan, Kay and I behaved pretty well in the backseat on most of those road trips. There were a few occasions, however, when things must have gotten out of hand. When verbal reprimands proved ineffective, Mother would resort to turning around with her removed shoe in hand and threaten to use it on all of us. I don't think she ever needed to.

Overall, there was little sibling rivalry between my sisters, brother and me. Since I was the youngest sister, I often tagged along with whichever older sister was available and feeling most tolerant. Once Susan trailblazed on into high school, she wasn't quite as accommodating. I was in awe of her for a long time. Besides being older, petite and thin, she got to do so many wonderful things first. She went out into the world getting that first paid babysitting job, got to wear makeup and was allowed to walk uptown on Friday night by herself to meet her friends. When she proudly strutted in front of Kay and me wearing her first pair of pantyhose and heels, we were both pretty darn envious. I wondered if such amazing things would ever happen for me.

Kay and I were almost inseparable, especially after Susan "outgrew" me, doing nearly everything together and always sharing a bedroom. We spent countless hours teaching our imaginary classrooms or playing with her friends, yes, I said her friends, at the park. Sometimes we did more crazy things like daring each other to walk around the edge of our old-fashioned, claw-legged bathtub without falling in, or worse, seeing how far we dared to climb up the town's water tower ladder. Mother would have been mortified. Kay was always the "doer." She could be counted on to get things done efficiently, correctly and on time. She was never late. I was never quite as organized or prepared as she was. I envied that about her. I still do.

Mark was five years younger than me, so he was mostly someone we had to look out for. We envied him for being a boy as well as the baby of the family. We knew even at our young ages the special advantages that position provided. He never had to share a bedroom, wear hand-me-downs or play with used toys.

I was the studious good girl. Good grades came easily for me, and I turned to writing early on as a way to express myself. I was quiet and pretty shy in public. It was terrifying for me on the few occasions when Kay was home sick without me, and I had to go into her classroom to pick up her homework. Luckily, that didn't happen very often because generally if one of us got sick, so did the other. We experienced measles, mumps and numerous bouts of strep throat and stomach flu together. We usually spent those sick days stretched out on the green couch in the dining room, one of us on each end.

The dining room of our house on Central Avenue North was quite large with plenty of room for a couch as well as a piano, desk and of course, the dining table that was positioned precisely in the center of the room. There was also a fireplace in the dining room, which impressed me and my siblings, even though for some reason we never used it other than as a background for holiday photos. That green couch was positioned to be in Mother's direct line of vision from the kitchen where she could keep a close eye on both of us while she tended to her work. She could determine just how sick we really were by how we were behaving on that green couch. If we appeared to be having too much fun, our sick days were over, and we were promptly sent back to school.

Even during Mother's illness, those long-established sibling positions somehow were still in place. Susan, living in Tennessee, still was someone far away and hard to get close to. Kay was still the "doer" and organizer, always ready with food and a schedule. Mark remained the highly prized son. I needed to be close to Mother and craved discussions and sharing. Those childhood qualities were pretty embedded in us, perhaps stemming from our birth order, but who really knows?

When mid-November arrived, I was once again back in Madelia to visit while Susan and Michael were there. They arrived looking fresh and rested, not tired and worn down like the rest of us. We took group pictures of all of us posing with Mother, as if trying to trap time in 4 x 6 photos. Later when I looked at them, I couldn't even tell she was sick. It looked like a typical family visit, but we all knew it was not.

Susan made salads, hot dishes and desserts and I wondered again how she still stayed so thin after all those years cooking meals with three courses. I never felt petite or thin enough for my family. Growing up I always felt different, awkward and out of place. Since sixth grade I've been taller than my sisters by half-a-foot, and complete strangers commented on this as if I didn't realize it myself.

How can you be the tallest if you are the youngest? That was the poorly thought-out question I heard countless times. It made me feel like being shorter would have been better. Mother, in her efforts to make me feel less self-conscious, quickly pointed out how she always wanted to be taller and what great advantages taller people had over shorter people, but somehow I couldn't figure out what those advantages were. As an awkward preteen, her words did not make me stand taller.

Even though Thanksgiving was still over two weeks away, we decided to put up the Christmas tree.

"We might as well put it up so Mother can enjoy something," Susan suggested.

I had to agree, so we lugged up plastic storage containers holding the tree and other decorations from the basement.

Thanksgiving arrived and Mother's appetite kept declining. Susan and Michael went back home to Tennessee, and I couldn't help thinking they were lucky to not have to face cancer close up every day like the rest of us. After convincing myself it would not make me a bad daughter, I decided to stay home and cook a Thanksgiving meal for my family in Wisconsin. Kay would have Thanksgiving dinner for her family, plus Mother, Dad and Mark. Kay lives on a hog farm minutes away from my parents' house so it would be convenient for them to get out there. At the end of the day I called her to see how things went.

"Mother only ate about a tablespoon of her favorites," Kay reported.

Watching a loved one's appetite decline during serious illness is one of the hardest parts to witness. Plus, food is such a part of who a mother is, a symbol representing all the nurturing they do. Most mothers put so much effort into food preparations for family events and celebrations, at least mine did. Mothers are sometimes even judged by what kind of cooks they are.

The Thanksgiving meal was one of Mother's best, and she proudly prepared it every year for whoever wanted to come. She always served the same things, and we rarely missed it. She knew it was my favorite meal and often prepared it for my birthday too. It tasted superb in February as well, but there was something about her turkey, mashed potatoes and gravy, stuffing and pumpkin pie served in late November that was truly worth anticipating all year long. Her only statement of defiance at Thanksgiving was refusing to get up early to "put the bird in the oven," as Dad used to say. My mother was not an early riser. She preferred to stay up late watching an old movie or reading a book and then sleep in the following morning.

The Friday after that Thanksgiving, my sons, Peter and Aaron, and I were on our way once again to Madelia. Peter was home from the University of North Dakota in Grand Forks and Aaron was a junior at Menomonie High School. They were eager to visit, but I was apprehensive because I knew there would be more decline in Mother's appearance and mood than they were prepared for. I was right. The rapid change was indeed unsettling and worrisome. That day she just wanted to sit in her La-Z-Boy recliner. She was unnaturally quiet, almost lethargic, and even sitting down she looked vulnerable and frail. She was not interested in reading, watching TV or even talking to her grandchildren. She was not herself.

I brought candles at that point whenever I visited even though I knew they were more for me than for her. Some unknown store clerk had told me lavender was supposed to be the most relaxing scent. So I brought a lavender one, as well as Mother's used-to-be favorites, cinnamon and rose petal. The sight and smell of gently burning candles did seem to be something she still enjoyed, and we were grateful for that. It was something.

Aaron made Grandma a personalized collection of CDs filled with a variety of music from Frank Sinatra to Simon and Garfunkel to his high school jazz pieces. Betty, her sister from Denver, sent countless cards and letters filled with words of encouragement and Francie, her other sister from Phoenix, called regularly. Mother was starting not to care much about our efforts, but we kept trying to plug up the invisible holes to keep cancer from flooding in over us.

Mother's friends kept calling to check on her, too, but often she didn't want to talk to them, so their calls became less frequent, as did their visits. I always felt a little envious of all the friends Mother had. She was much better at making friends than me. She was outgoing and seemed to accumulate quite a few. Now this woman who had always loved friends and conversation so much seemed to avoid both. There wasn't enough time or energy to spare anymore. Conversation was becoming too cumbersome a task. Her world was shrinking daily.

Shit.

Why was our wonder drug not working?

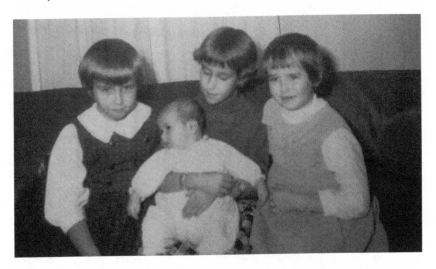

Posing with my siblings in the living room of our house on Central Avenue North. That's Kay, Susan holding Mark, and me on the far right.

-11-

May Just Sucks

May 1

I have almost no more soreness or tenderness left from the biopsy, but my left breast looks bruised with various shades of green, blue and deep purple around the site. I tell David to look at it so he can begin to get used to seeing such things. I'm not sure what sights are ahead, but I know things will look worse than this. Much worse.

This afternoon I am busy Googling away, gathering information about lumpectomies, mastectomies and reconstruction. I didn't realize there were so many variations for the latter two. I research and begin to comprehend. I feel nauseous and decide I need to slow down. The sick feeling soon passes as I once again absorb pieces of information which might represent my future. I cannot allow my mind to be flooded too quickly with all of cancer's frightening challenges. I must let such things trickle in more slowly or I will drown in the overwhelming uncertainty of it all.

May 3

Last night I slept better than I have in a week, and I wake up refreshed and recharged by sleep's healing powers. A rested mind definitely copes better, thinks more clearly, feels more invincible, generates more optimistic thoughts and is far more pleasant to be around. David notices my upbeat mood and I'm sure is happy for a good start to the day.

I head back to the mall to purchase some newly decided upon necessities. The first is a down pillow. It's priced at $120 at Macy's. I've never spent so much on a pillow, but suddenly paying this price to potentially help me get a good night's sleep seems totally reasonable, maybe even necessary.

Next I head to the lingerie department to pick out some pajamas with button-down tops. Someone like me who will soon be having a lumpectomy or a bilateral mastectomy will require button-down pajama tops, will I not? Actually, I have no idea what I'll need. Ironically, Macy's is celebrating breast cancer research something or other, and the clerk hands me a pink ribbon as I enter the dressing room. What the heck? It's not even October. Breast Cancer Awareness Month is still months from now. A bra-fitting event is also taking place with a specialist available to measure and fit me for a proper-fitting bra. Maybe I picked the wrong day to shop.

"Do you have any interest in being fitted today?" the clerk asks.

"No thank you," I say.

There is no need to measure my chest. In a short while I may no longer even have breasts. At least she couldn't tell by looking at me I have cancer.

The day's final necessity is a new purse. There is no particular reason or requirement, but I have determined today I will buy one. I carefully survey them all, studying their sizes, shapes and colors, hidden pockets and zippers as if I am making some highly important decision. Ironically, I decide on a pink one.

Tonight David and I continue our pretend, almost jovial, mood. We must be in cancer denial mode or something. We take our two-mile walk, eat dinner, mindlessly watch *M*A*S*H* reruns and even joke about breast implants. When he gets up from his comfortable, leather recliner to go to bed, once again I am in tears. Immediately he feels badly for joking about such things, and I try to explain it's nothing he said. Suddenly I am simply feeling overwhelmed. But no words that make sense find their way out of my mouth. I am unsuccessful at making him understand my fear and loneliness. Who could? I don't even understand these things myself. I wonder if he cries, too, when I cannot see.

May 4

The $120 down pillow experiment is a failure.

May 7

I have officially had cancer for one week, but who knows how long it's actually been lurking and growing in my body. There is another doctor appointment today. I am already sick of doctor appointments, and there are so many ahead. I can't think about that. I must focus on today's appointment, the one with a plastic surgeon.

I never thought I would need an appointment with a plastic surgeon. I would not be one of those women afraid to age. I would not succumb to facelifts, tummy tucks, liposuction, BOTOX or anti-aging agents making unkeepable promises. Not me. I would age gracefully and allow nature to take its course. I never even thought about needing a plastic surgeon for other reasons, like cancer and breast reconstruction. Such possibilities had never entered my mind.

Being in a plastic surgeon's exam room feels unfathomable for a lot of reasons, but this is where I find myself today. David and I must begin to prepare for worst-case scenarios. We must prepare for mastectomies and reconstructed breasts. These "options" are what will be recommended if my BRCA2 gene mutation test comes back positive. Bilateral mastectomy, even the words sound daunting and forebodingly horrendous. We are here today to discuss reconstruction. Reconstruction sounds like something you do to a major highway or a building, not your breasts.

The plastic surgeon's name is Dr. Banich. He is pleasant and nice enough but unable to make me feel comfortable. I'm not sure anyone could. He apologizes for not being more familiar with my case, which I again must explain in detail. I am uneasy and nervous, feeling my face becoming hot and red from embarrassment. My neck and chest break out with a red, blotchy-looking rash.

We discuss various reconstruction options and finally zero in on the implant one. Dr. Banich rummages through a drawer and pulls out implant samples made of clear plastic of some sort and filled with silicone, a clear-looking, thick gel. No wonder they're sometimes referred to as Gummy Bears. We pass around the sample "breasts" squeezing and squishing them, all of us pretending replacing my real breasts with them will be no big deal. He explains the reconstruction process, bringing reality into the picture.

My surgery will be a team effort. The first step, the bilateral mastectomy, will be done by a different surgeon. The plastic surgeon does not remove breasts; he only builds new ones. After removal of my originals, then, and only then, he will step in, put in place temporary tissue expanders, fill them a bit (so I would at least have *something* there, he says) and then skillfully stitch me up, hoping for minimal scarring that should fade somewhat in time. I will need to return every few weeks or so to keep filling the tissue expanders slowly over time. Their temporary job, more or less, will be to keep a space ready for my eventual, more permanent, silicone replacements. Those will have to wait until chemo is over, if I should need it, and I hope to God I will not.

Reconstruction is a process which continues in steps taken over several months. We now fully realize this will not be quick or easy. You don't reconstruct breasts overnight.

"In the end, I think you will be quite satisfied with the results," Dr. Banich says.

He correctly senses we are feeling overwhelmed.

Next, I stand with my bare chest directly in front of his eyes as he sits on his stool in front of me. He takes out his tape measure and begins measuring and calculating in order to estimate my proper size. What a peculiar way to make a living, I think to myself. Finally, that humiliation is over, and we go over our numerous questions as nonchalantly as possible.

"Yes, you are a good candidate for reconstruction," he says. "I can definitely help you, if you choose to go this route."

This is good news. Our idea about what constitutes good news is drastically altered. Plus, I like how he said it's my choice. Maybe he's not so bad after all.

As we wrap up our meeting, his nurse comes back into the room with a camera for God's sake. She escorts me to another room where I stand topless in front of a blue screen like the kind kids pose in front of for their annual school pictures. She gives me directions about how to stand and turn, which I robotically follow. My breasts are photographed, preserved for study and comparison, suddenly specimens requiring digital documentation. They are now originals for which copies must be made. I know it is silly, but I feel awkward, exposed, embarrassed and even a little cheap.

I wonder where David is and what he is thinking about while he waits. What will he really think the first time he sees his wife without breasts? How will he feel? How will I feel? How bad will I look? Will I ever look attractive to him again? How will he really feel when he empties my drain tubes?

When I return and see his face, I know he is worried and concerned, but not about these things. Once again I feel grateful someone loves me this much, with or without breasts. As we leave the exam room and head for the elevators, we both breathe easier. Somehow we know we can make it.

Mother's Day Weekend

It's the Saturday before Mother's Day and I should be in a good mood, but I am an emotional mess. I have another crying episode, not the quiet, almost unnoticeable kind, but the type where I wail, making unpleasant, almost unrecognizable noises. I am frustrated and just plain miserable. This latest round is set off by a seemingly innocent comment David makes while we are driving around. Such a comment would not normally bother me, but today my tears are unexplainable, quick to spill out and unstoppable. All I can do is grab my sunglasses despite the fact it is cloudy and attempt to hide behind them.

Later when we get home and I am alone, I find myself continuing to sob. I am hurt, angry, disgusted and outraged, not with David, but with my situation, with myself.

David leaves. I think he needs to get away from me for a while. I can't blame him. I'm hard to be around these days.

Finally, I pull myself together, take a shower and realize I can't expect David to never get annoyed or even angry with me simply because I have cancer. I don't even want such a thing. I do not want to be treated differently. I'm a basket case.

Lindsay and her boyfriend Josh arrive this afternoon from Fargo, North Dakota. There is nothing to eat in the house, so we decide to have an early dinner out at a Chinese place. Everyone complains about the food and insists it was no good, but I thought everything tasted fine. Why am I so disagreeable about everything, even Chinese food?

When we get home, we sit around outside on lawn chairs watching the dogs. Ace (Lindsay's dog), Elsie and Sophie run around retrieving sticks and balls over and over again. We play Monopoly. No one mentions cancer. Things feel awkward and weird.

When I finally go to bed, I'm exhausted. My eyes still feel dry from my earlier crying jag and lack of sleep. I am eager to go to bed. I pull the covers over my face and for once, I fall asleep immediately.

It was really sweet of Lindsay and Josh to come visit me for Mother's Day. Still, having people around, even my own family is hard, too, and I wonder what the summer will be like when Peter and Aaron are home. I feel like I must maintain my motherly role around my kids, even though they aren't even kids anymore. I don't want them to see me vulnerable, weak and weepy. I know it's silly, but knowing so doesn't make me stop thinking this way.

On Mother's Day we do discuss my cancer and I'm glad. We do it while lingering over coffee. We discuss appointments, gene tests, options and surgeries. We focus on concrete things, not personal, emotional stuff because that's way harder. I wonder how worried Lindsay really is. Does she envision me ending up like Grandma? Does she worry about getting cancer herself? Does she think I look too tired and worried? Why don't I just ask her these things? Why is everything so hard?

When it's time for Lindsay and Josh to leave, I take pictures of them standing in front of the blooming crab apple tree we planted last summer, before cancer. It's covered with beautiful, deep pink blossoms. We say goodbye and I watch them drive away. They drive away from me. They drive away from cancer.

I decide to lie down and take a rest where I can see the pine trees from the window in my bedroom. A few boats go by on the little lake we live on, but it's pretty quiet. Other families are busy celebrating Mother's Day in homes without cancer. I wait for David to join me, but he doesn't. I could ask him to come, but that seems too needy. I hear him sleeping, snoring actually, from the recliner in the other room. Is he avoiding me? Is he pulling away already?

After we have both rested, we get ready to go to Aaron's choir concert at the University in Eau Claire. When Aaron walks onto the stage, he looks so grown up, mature and handsome wearing his black suit we recently bought him. When he sings, he looks so happy, and I'm grateful he has this gift of music in his life. I love watching him sing.

"You are the best looking woman here," David says unexpectedly and for no reason at all during intermission.

I immediately feel guilty for my earlier thoughts.

"Yeah, right," I answer.

"Just look around, I'm a lucky bastard," he says.

He is joking, but he is serious too.

I guess he isn't pulling away. I am lucky. Despite cancer, I am still a lucky woman. I guess it's been a good Mother's Day weekend after all.

May 10

I substitute in third grade today, and boy it feels good to hang out all day with a bunch of eight and nine-year-olds who treat me like an ordinary substitute teacher. They are oblivious to cancer worries and concerns. I wonder how many of their families have been snared by cancer's tentacles. They act like normal kids and do normal kid things. The ordinariness of a third-grade classroom on an ordinary Monday in May feels like something special. It reminds me cancer does not define me, not totally anyway. It is only a fraction of who I am. I am a teacher, someone who makes a difference every day. Take *that*, cancer!

May 12

I wait for the phone call to give me the result of my gene test, but my phone remains silent even though I keep looking at it, as if willing it to ring. The waiting is getting harder. I want to get on to the next phase, the treatment phase, but yet I do not. I want to hide here in this mysterious limbo-of-not-knowing phase. It feels like none of this is really happening to me. Nothing has changed, yet everything has changed. I will never be the same person I was again.

David and I meet with yet another doctor. I am so sick of doctor appointments already. They make me feel like I am sick and I feel fine. How can I feel fine if I have cancer? I am not fine.

This time we meet with the surgeon who will literally change my life. His name is Dr. Hower, and luckily both David and I like him a lot. He seems very knowledgeable, obviously likes to talk and seems genuinely concerned. As we discuss my options, I contemplate how the course of my life is literally in his surgeon hands. He will be the one to remove my breasts if I am BRCA2 positive. Or, the lesser of two evils may happen, and he will simply carve out a portion of my left breast. I have two options and I don't like either one. Of course the third option is to do nothing, but then I die. It would only be a matter of time. What kind of options are these?

He explains both scenarios in careful detail answering each question we come up with. He doesn't make us feel like we have too many. I'm grateful for his patience.

"How bad will I look after a bilateral mastectomy?" I blurt out.

Dr. Hower must think I'm a very vain person. How can I be worrying about how I will look? I should be worrying about dying.

"Will David be able to handle the drain tubes?"

It's another stupid question that tumbles out of my mouth. Somehow Dr. Hower doesn't seem to think these questions are odd at all.

"No, you will not look bad, and David will be just fine," he says.

Dr. Hower is a very compassionate human being, not just a compassionate doctor, a compassionate human being.

"Don't worry about that part," David says.

But I do. How can I not? What will he really think the first time he see me?

After the majority of our discussion concludes, this doctor too must examine me, and I make a mental tally of how many doctors and nurses have now peered at and palpitated my breasts. The number keeps growing. Dr. Hower shows me where the incisions will be made for either procedure. His hands feel like surgeon hands. They move slowly and carefully.

By the time David and I leave the clinic it is almost 6 p.m., and the place is eerily quiet since almost everyone has left for the day. Everyone has gone home to their cancer-free lives. Even the lights have been turned off. I can hardly wait to get home and sink myself into my familiar and comfortable blue, leather sofa. It has become my sofa. It has become my place to absorb, analyze, process, rant, cry, rest, journal, mindlessly watch TV, lounge, sleep and just be. It's only a piece of furniture, but it feels like a sofa haven, a liferaft of sorts in these unsettled waters of cancer. I feel safe on my blue, leather sofa. I float.

May 14

Today is my last day to substitute this school year. I can't take any assignments next week or the week after that because I don't know what the hell I'll be doing. I can't plan anything it seems other than more appointments. I am ready to get my surgery over with, whatever kind I must have.

No gene test results yet. I call the clinic to check, just to be sure they haven't forgotten about me. The nurse reassures me they have not. It's Friday afternoon and I am convinced the results are in, but she's making me wait until Monday. Why don't I believe her?

May 17

It's the start of a new week and with it comes more waiting. It's been four weeks since the mass sighting. Four fucking weeks!

I hate the waiting, yet I love and welcome the waiting. I want to know what is ahead, yet I do not. While I am waiting, I get to remain normal. I keep doing normal things, almost floating through the days in semi-consciousness. Sometimes I must remind myself I have cancer because it seems so impossible and nothing has really changed yet. Then I realize everything has changed, and I cannot pretend or deny much longer. My waiting phase is about over, and then I must step into the action phase, the phase where I must treat the breast cancer beast if I want to live.

I feel unrealistically safe in the waiting phase. I am not safe. I am frightened and overwhelmed when I think about the action phase. It's too daunting and full of uncertainty. I tell myself thousands of other women have gone through what I now face. Why should I think I am special? Why should other women get breast cancer and not me? Why should I be immune? If other women have handled their cancers, shouldn't I be able to? Shouldn't this knowledge give me confidence? It doesn't.

Some days I do feel confident and capable, and some days I do not feel capable of handling much at all. Some days I cry too many times to count, and some days I don't shed a single tear. All my feelings, worries and questions are normal for someone in my position, I keep hearing and reading. Normal, normal, normal. I am now a woman who has breast cancer. What kind of normal is this?

May 18

I feel like we now have a sign staked in my front yard like the ones politicians and campaigns erect to promote their candidate. Only instead of displaying some candidate's name, my sign says, *Nancy Stordahl lives here and she has breast cancer.* It seems as if everyone who drives by can see this is where someone with cancer lives. This is totally ridiculous. Of course it isn't true, and even if it were, no one would give a damn. Am I becoming paranoid too?

I'm invited to coffee at a neighbor's house today, and I go reluctantly because now I have to tell my story again. I can't keep truth plugged up; it's slowly leaking out.

"I have some news and it's not good news," I blurt out while sipping coffee and nibbling on a piece of some kind of gooey pastry. "I have breast cancer."

Well, how on earth are people supposed to respond to that? All eyes uneasily shift in my direction, and I insert my story into the previously lighthearted conversation like an out-of-place chapter in a book. They try to be sympathetic and supportive, but they don't comprehend. No one can.

Luckily I get to leave early because lo and behold, I have another doctor appointment this morning. This will be my second appointment with my oncologist. My gene test results are in.

Dr. Nambudiri slowly enters the room carrying the purple folder. The BRCA test results come back in a purple folder. I remember this from Mother's test. At least it's not pink.

"Your test was positive," Dr. Nambudiri says.

He opens the purple folder and once again, there it is in dark bold print as if further emphasizing my doom, positive for a **deleterious mutation.** Again, I think it sounds more like some mental illness. So there it is. The words have been said out loud somehow amplifying their power and significance. We aren't surprised really. We have begun to anticipate worst-case scenarios by now.

Dr. Nambudiri seems kinder and more compassionate today, after all, he is delivering more bad news. My patient status has moved up a notch, or down, depending upon how you look at it. Now my treatment options aren't really options at all. Now a bilateral mastectomy is the only one I'm supposed to consider, if I want to increase my odds of living. I do want to. Dr. Nambudiri brings up statistics on his computer screen where such things as surgery, hormone therapy and chemo are depicted in brightly colored blue, yellow and green bar graphs, each capable of adding percentage points onto my survival odds. My life expectancy is now some sort of crapshoot, and we're weighing all the odds trying to best figure out where to place our bets. Bilateral mastectomy it will be. It's time to make arrangements.

"We'll get through this together. It'll be alright," David says.

He puts his arm around me because he sees I am struggling to hold myself together.

Only a couple tears manage to escape as I will myself to hold it together. I must not crumble in this place. I will not.

Once back home, I spend the rest of the afternoon fluctuating between crying rampages and downright ugly anger outbursts. I know David feels uncomfortable when I cry, but I can't stop and I don't care. I feel so alone. This is my body and these are my breasts. This is my cancer. I'm not alone but yet I am.

Finally, I start pulling myself together when my phone rings. I hand it to David feeling cowardly, weak, vulnerable and unable to even accept a freaking phone call. It's Dr. Hower calling to schedule my surgery date. I hear David say June 2 will be fine. What the fuck? How can June 2 be fine? June 2 is two more weeks away! How am I supposed to sit around waiting for two more weeks? It's already been four. I flee from the family room feeling sick to my stomach.

"Is this the best they can do?" I plead from the next room.

I am forced to comply with the hospital's and the surgeon's time-table. They don't feel hurried like I do. I have no say, or so it seems. Again, I am sobbing and acting irrationally, and I know it. I am disgusting, impatient, angry and unreasonable. I need to get a grip, but I don't know how to. I don't have a clue.

"I need to go to the office for a while to check on some things," David says.

It's 4 p.m. in the afternoon for crying out loud, and he finally leaves for work. He must be glad to get out of the house. He must be glad to get away from me, away from cancer, even if only for a few hours. I would be.

The day finally ends and I am exhausted. This has been one of the worst days of my life, worse than the day of the mass sighting, worse than the day that idiot doctor told me I had "a" cancer. I wonder if there are worse yet days to come. There are.

May 21-22

Today David and I are driving to Fargo, where we will walk in the 10K which is part of the larger Fargo Marathon annual event. We feel excited to face this challenge and diversion from cancer, even if it's only for a few hours. The five-hour drive along I-94 goes by quickly as we have much to talk about. I wonder if David gets sick of talking about cancer. He must because I surely do, yet it seems we can't focus on much else, at least not for very long. I think of all the times I have driven on this particular highway, all the times when I was cancer free.

Tonight we take Lindsay and Josh out to dinner and talk about biopsies, co-payments, surgeries and drugs. It feels like we are talking about another person, not me. As evening closes in, David and I are anxious to return to our motel room to rest our minds and bodies.

"Do you want to come over and hang out some more?" Lindsay asks.

I try to explain our exhaustion and desire to be alone, but I don't think I'm very successful.

David and I collapse into bed. Minutes later we are acting like a couple of newlyweds, as if experiencing intimacy is new to us. I am mentally calculating the days and hours until my body is carved up, and I am no longer physically the person he married.

"Don't be afraid to touch my breasts," I say. "I have to remember what it feels like."

The surgeon's words fill my mind, the ones about no more feeling after a bilateral. I must store up such memories. I must remember. I must not forget. Tears stream down my face in the darkness, and I wonder if David notices. If he does, he doesn't mention it. He must store up the memories too.

The morning news brings with it a turbulent weather forecast. I look out the window to check, but it's still dark. It's only 4:30 a.m. Turbulent weather for turbulent times; it seems to fit.

Eventually 7 a.m. arrives and the 10K is underway. David and I surge forward blending into the nameless faces of the crowd. It feels wonderful to blend in, to be so invisible. Lindsay and Josh are somewhere behind, but soon they catch up and pass us. The drizzle turns to rain and we spend the next hour and 45 minutes or so sloshing through puddles, following arrows, encouraging each other, talking and immersing ourselves into the experience as if walking in the rain will wash away the cancer. The cold rain cleanses us, and we aren't even shivering. For this short time we are part of something else, and no one knows I have cancer.

We cross the finish line, but we know many others of a much different kind are ahead. We hope we can cross those too.

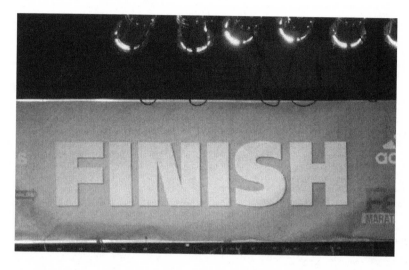

Finishing the Fargo Marathon 10K just days before my bilateral was something I had to do. It was symbolic in some way I guess.

-12-

One More Christmas

As we walked through the cancer wing after entering the hospital for yet another doctor appointment for Mother, we passed the chapel strategically placed for easy access near the cancer area, but it was empty. I noticed hand sanitizer pumps were everywhere so hospital visitors, staff and patients could wash away germs, but nothing can wash away cancer. I was beginning to lose track of how many appointments we had been to. December had arrived, so a Christmas tree had been added in the waiting room looking too small, too blue and too artificial. It was tucked away in the corner and had no decorations, almost as if trying to not look too festive.

A nurse wearing a blue uniform, a Christmas pin and candy cane earrings checked Mother's weight and reported she had lost another five pounds. We sat down to wait for her name to be called while looking for someone who appeared sicker to walk through the door. If we saw sicker people walk through the door, then we knew we had more time, but not much more.

When we got to the exam room, a different nurse took Mother's vitals and asked the usual questions.

"Can you rate the pain and nausea you are feeling today on a scale of one to ten with ten being the highest?" the nurse asked.

"Oh, my pain's about a five," Mother said.

Immediately I started squirming because I knew darn well it was higher than that. Why did she always minimize her pain when we got there? And why did this annoy me so much?

"I think it's really at least a seven," I blurted out.

What I really wanted to say was, why in the world can't you help her? Your stupid scale is worthless if you can't help her. Of course, such things were not possible to say out loud.

Her oncologist finally appeared wearing a wrinkled, black suit and his thin, reddish-blond hair was uncombed. He looked as if he was always in a hurry rushing from one cancer patient to the next. He probably rushed home at night, too, without taking time to properly hang up his suit. He looked uncomfortable, probably because he knew he had nothing to say that we wanted to hear. I was beginning to find him disappointing.

"I can't understand why your mother is so nauseous," he said. "No one should be this nauseous, even someone with cancer like hers. I have never seen anyone else experience such a bad case of it."

He was baffled and kept repeating this over and over as if doing so would make us feel better. It didn't. Instead his comments felt patronizing and unhelpful, and I was losing my tolerance for the guy.

A day later I was back home in Wisconsin getting ready for the holidays which felt undoable. I was going through the motions, as if watching another person making all the preparations that other years seemed so necessary. That year I had too many other things on my mind, mostly preparing for my last Christmas as a daughter with a mother.

Christmas had always been such a happy time, definitely Mother's favorite holiday. She always went way out, okay, overboard. The baking would begin right after Thanksgiving and sometimes before. Krumkake and rosettes were always the first things made.

When I was growing up, I was often recruited to assist with these two jobs. Both are made with extremely hot irons, and the process for both always scared me a little. Krumkake is a Norwegian treat made by dropping a teaspoon full of creamy, buttery dough onto a very hot two-sided griddle which you then squeeze together and rotate over a hot burner until the golden-brown circle is plopped out onto the counter and immediately rolled into a scroll before it cools. If you wait too long, you cannot roll it into the proper configuration and you have to try again. A lot of timing, coordination, quickness and patience is required, not to mention, tough fingers.

Rosettes, also a delicate Scandinavian delight, were easier for the assistant anyway. All I had to do was roll the finished product around in some sugar. Rosettes were deep fried in hot oil, and that part always frightened me, especially when an occasional flame shot up off the burner when some oil was inadvertently dripped. Mother calmly put out any such flare-ups with a pot lid she kept close by.

Mother's krumkake and rosettes were famous in Madelia and instantly sold out each year at the annual church bazaar for which she and her assistant also created these specialties. No other occasions warranted krumkake and rosette making. Christmas and the annual church bazaar were the only two.

Sugar cookies were next on the to do list and Mother knew how to make the perfect sugar cookie, which required rolling the dough out as thinly as possible.

"The thinner the better," she would say. "The perfect sugar cookie must be thin, crisp and a delicate golden brown."

Some of my friends' mothers made thick, chewy sugar cookies, but I always knew they were not the perfect sugar cookies like my mother's were.

Every holiday season a wide variety of other goodies would also appear, but there was never a year without krumkake, rosettes and sugar cookies. Eventually the time came for them to be taken out of the freezer or cupboard hiding place, and they would all be beautifully displayed on crystal trays. Mother carefully rationed them out each year to make sure they lasted until Susan's birthday on January 2.

Somehow amongst all the baking frenzy, the house would get decorated from top to bottom, and of course, there was shopping. And more shopping. By Christmas Eve the gifts were piled so high they wouldn't even fit under the tree anymore.

On that Christmas Eve Mark called with upsetting news.

"It's in her liver now and probably other places too," he said.

He didn't need to say much else. We all knew what it meant. Mother's disease was progressing, but even more importantly, it was doing so at an incredibly rapid speed, as if it were in some sort of race to the finish line. Even her doctors were surprised. We needed a new plan and we needed it soon.

I was ashamed of myself for feeling irritated with Mark. Why did they schedule an appointment on Christmas Eve? Who does that? You aren't supposed to get bad news on Christmas Eve. We were just about to open gifts for heaven's sake.

"I thought you would want to know right away," Mark said.

Of course, he was right. Still the new information was overwhelming, and I struggled to hold back most of my tears, waiting to share the news with the rest of my family until we were finished opening gifts. Another special day was forever tarnished by cancer.

Despite bad news, Christmas Day arrived, ready for it or not. David, Peter, Aaron and I traveled to Madelia to spend one last Christmas with Mother. In thirty years, David and I had missed that holiday trip to Madelia only twice. When we were newlyweds, we took a trip to Arizona and California over Christmas and didn't make it. The other time was when Lindsay was an infant and sick with a high fever from an ear infection. That year we made a trip to the emergency room on Christmas Day instead, but even then we only postponed our Madelia trip for one day. It's not that we didn't want to be home on Christmas Day every year; we did. However, I'm sure there were a few years when travel was hazardous, and staying home might have been the more sensible option. But disappointing Mother at Christmas was out of the question.

My last Christmas with a mother was very different, surreal in fact.

"She's just not eating anything," my dad said.

That was the Christmas greeting I received even before I had made it through the front door. Dad was now obsessed with how much Mother was eating or not eating and judged how she was doing accordingly.

Dad and Mark had done their best decorating and trying to make the place look festive, but cancer loomed everywhere, almost a tangible presence lurking in the very air we breathed. There was a fire in the gas fireplace, the usual fruity punch Kay makes with orange juice, pineapple juice and 7UP ready to serve up from Mother's punch bowl, the glowing Christmas tree that looked like it was too quickly decorated and the usual gathering of relatives; but all I saw and felt was cancer. Mandi, my parents' cairn terrier, and Radar, were bouncing around happily playing with pieces of wrapping paper, enjoying the extra commotion and attention they were getting.

I noticed the noise and activity of opening gifts, barking dogs and excited voices seemed to be bothering Mother. That was a stark contrast to years gone by when the more people and noise there was, the happier she would be. She had always loved the excitement a full house of grandchildren brought, even the boisterous misbehaving which inevitably happened each year seemed to delight her. On that last Christmas, she made attempts at conversation and opened her gifts with slow-moving, uncooperative hands. Kay and I were unable to talk her into sampling even a cookie or piece of fudge. We were all going through the motions of eating and gift opening, but there was no realness to any of it, and I was relieved when we were done pretending. Pretending felt pointless, even on Christmas.

Later that December, one of my nephews was getting married. Normally Mother would have been bubbling with excitement and enthusiasm for such an event. She planned a December wedding before. Mine.

I've always thought December was the perfect month for a wedding, so of course, that's the month David and I chose to get married. We picked December 18, right smack in the middle of the regular holiday frenzy. I'm sure my parents were running around frantically that year, but selfishly, I suppose, I never noticed. The church looked like a Christmas card that night with candles burning in the windows, Christmas lights and the smell of evergreen in the air from the fresh-cut greenery adorning the pews. My mother had made sure everything was perfect. And it was.

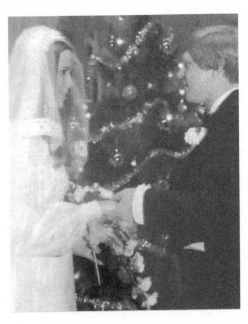

Our magical December wedding

For my nephew's wedding, I sat in a pew at the back of the un-familiar church in Mankato, Minnesota, waiting for Mother, Dad and Mark to arrive. They showed up minutes before the ceremony was about to start. Mark was carefully pushing Mother in a wheelchair, and Dad was following close behind looking unsure of what he should be doing. The sight took my breath away, and I wanted to cry, but I could not allow that. I didn't want to spoil a wedding. *I would not spoil a wedding.* I wondered what the rest of the family was thinking. Why did they all look so poised and normal? Seeing the new unwelcome development of the wheelchair was shocking even though I knew it was coming. It was a cruel, visual reminder we really were living the nightmare. I felt badly for Kay and her family, unfairly having to juggle feelings of happiness and sadness at an occasion where there should only be joy.

Mother looked nice all dressed up, with her hair done and wearing a grandmother corsage pinned to her lapel. She stayed solemn and quiet putting up with our insistence of including her in too many pictures with various family members. Following the ceremony, we tried to be festive at our reception table as we sat surrounded by glowing white Christmas lights and dozens of red poinsettias. It all looked so lovely, and I tried to smile so I, too, would fit in with the loveliness. But I did not fit in.

"Don't put much on my plate," Mother begged of me when I got in line to get her food.

After we finished eating, I walked around talking to people with a fake smile, pretending to feel fine while explaining the wheelchair development. It was a lovely wedding, but I was relieved when it ended, and we could all just go home and stop pretending.

-13-

Countdown to No Breasts

May 26 – one week

It's only one more week until my surgery. I have one more week to have breasts, my breasts. I must be vain and silly to be focusing so much on losing my breasts when instead I should be focusing on ridding my body of cancer and staying alive, but I can't help it. I can't stop wondering about the new image I will soon be seeing when I look in the mirror. I have no clue what that image will look like, but I imagine it to be something quite unpleasant.

This afternoon David and I meet again with my general surgeon, Dr. Hower. Nurse Dwayne checks us in and talks about his two dogs. I like Dwayne, but it's still hard to accept the fact so many men are allowed to become familiar with my chest.

When Dr. Hower enters the exam room, he immediately walks over to me, smiles and shakes my hand.

"Are you doing okay? You look good," he says.

Why do doctors ask you if you are okay? Clearly cancer patients are not okay. Someone should tell them to think of something else to say. He proceeds to carefully explain my upcoming surgery. He makes marks and notes on diagrams he draws. He takes time to answer all our questions and offers genuine reassurance.

"You'll be fine," he says.

Another thing maybe doctors shouldn't say, but I almost believe him. I want to believe him.

May 27 – six days

Today I am on my way to Madelia since Susan has arrived from Tennessee to visit Dad. I feel nervous about my visit. I remember my last trip to Madelia. That was when my "heart attack" symptoms kicked into high gear. Also, I have to face my family, and I know we will all be uncomfortable. I decide to take Sophie along. She will be good company as well as a distraction.

When Sophie and I arrive, we go immediately to the backyard because it's a nice day, and I know everyone will be outside sitting on Dad's patio. Dad and Kay are sitting on lawn chairs and my niece, Rachel, is there with her fiancé.

"Hello, Nancy," Rachel says.

I wonder if she is really glad to see me or just pretending.

Susan is in the kitchen preparing food, and the smells of freshly baked quiche, cheesy potatoes and coffee make their way out to the backyard. Suddenly I realize I'm ravenous.

We spend the entire afternoon outdoors. Mark arrives with Radar and another dog he is pet sitting. Kay's dog Daisy is here, too, as well as Mandi, so with five dogs there is plenty of activity. We sit around in the company of our uninvited guest, cancer. Dad looks tired. It must be hard to have a daughter with cancer. Is it worse than having a wife with cancer?

"Well, how did your appointment go yesterday?" Kay asks as she sits down next to me.

I'm relieved someone is finally going to talk about things. I explain the details of my surgery, reconstruction, pathology report and possible outcomes as completely but yet as briefly as I am able. I feel guilty for making my family deal with cancer again so soon after Mother's. I brought the dark cloud back too soon. They try not to look at me differently. They try to treat me the same. But I'm not the same.

When it's time to go home, there are more awkward hugs. They will be thinking of me, they say. Sophie and I pull out of the driveway, and I still look for Mother, almost expecting to see her standing on the porch waving. Instead, all I see is that empty space where she is supposed to be standing. I miss her. I feel a strong desire to get home, back to David, back to my house, back to my blue, leather sofa, back to things that feel familiar and safe.

Sophie is worn out from the warm day and from running around with the other dogs. She sleeps curled up on the passenger seat next to me, hardly moving for three hours. Once in a while she opens her eyes to check on me, and I give her an occasional pat on the head. I drive. I listen to mindless talk shows on the radio. They talk about problems but offer few solutions. Except for a few patches of traffic and road construction, the drive is peaceful and enjoyable. Cars whisk past me, and I wonder if any of them hold people who have cancer. As dusk and darkness slowly overtake the daylight creating a lovely transition into evening, my mind slows down as well, making a kind of transition of its own. Today was a difficult day. Today was also a good day. I know more of both are ahead.

May 29 – four days

I am grieving for my breasts. Maybe that sounds odd, I don't know, but I've decided that's what I'm doing. I've probably been grieving for the healthy body I no longer have since the day in the ER room, the day of the mass sighting.

Most women are not entirely happy or satisfied with their bodies, and I am no exception. Mine, too, is flawed and full of imperfections. As a young girl, I always felt too tall, but in reality the rest of my family was short. I towered over my mother and sisters always feeling out of place. I was never strong or athletic, merely getting by in gym class. I dreaded everything about gym class, from the incredibly ugly one-piece, royal-blue uniform to the dark, dreary, damp locker room, to the humiliation I often ended up feeling due to my inadequate abilities to jump a hurdle, do a cartwheel or throw a softball far enough. Luckily, I had loyal friends who never deserted me when it came time for picking teams. The best thing about my junior and senior years of high school was the fact there was no more gym class with Mrs. Nelson, a nice enough teacher, but one who didn't have a lot of time or patience for the non-athletic type like me.

Later on as an adult, I grew to appreciate my body's strengths. There's nothing like experiencing three normal pregnancies and giving birth three times to make you realize your body is pretty darn miraculous after all. I was finally comfortable with my height and strong body, even if it had a few extra pounds, some unsightly veins and had difficulty maintaining good posture due to all those years of "being too tall." I felt more at peace and confident with each passing decade. I assumed I would remain healthy and strong. I was certainly not expecting my body to betray me and to hear the words, you have cancer. How did this happen?

Yes, I am grieving for the loss of not only my breasts I am about to lose, but also for a complete and whole, healthy body. And a long life is in question now too, another thing to grieve for.

David doesn't entirely understand this grieving for breasts.

"You have cancer in one of them, and the risk is too great for cancer to appear in the other one to keep it," he reminds me again today. "If you keep your breasts, you will die. It's that simple."

But it isn't.

I know he is right. My breasts have never been all that great, they're not my best feature, but they are mine. I don't want to give them up, and I am grieving for this loss that I know is coming.

May 30 – three days

Three more days until my surgery, and this is counting today. There are only three more days before they amputate my breasts. This is what it should be called, an amputation, because this is what it feels like it is to me. Why are we all so breast-obsessed anyway? Clumps of fatty tissue anywhere else on a woman's body are despised, aren't they? What is so special about breasts?

I have a really good day today crossing things off my to do list, spending time outside in my yard and flower gardens, watching the dogs run around and trying to relax. Tonight David and Aaron decide to settle in to watch a movie. I attempt to join them and try to focus in on it, too, even though I have no interest. Almost immediately I am fidgety and bored with TV movies. I'm annoyed with a husband and son who want to watch one, but I say nothing. They are both smiling and laughing, obviously engaged in some stupid movie. They are being normal. How is this possible? This is not a normal evening before another normal day. I leave the room, and they don't notice or else they pretend not to. I make a lame attempt to journal and then read in another room, but I am unsuccessful at both. I decide to go get ready for bed.

After a few minutes have passed, David comes to look for me.

"What's wrong?" he asks.

Instantly, of course, the tears start flowing. He understands and puts his arms around me, but this makes me cry harder.

"Just lie down," he says.

He puts on a relaxing CD and then lies down next to me. As abruptly as they began, my tears subside. I begin to relax finding comfort in the loving arms of my husband and in the soothing veil of dusk as well.

Lindsay calls and again the tears come, but it doesn't matter. She is now a daughter who has a mother with cancer. Her life is changed too. My children shouldn't have to have a mother with cancer. Not yet.

I am exhausted. I close my eyes and try to sleep. There is no cancer when I sleep.

June 1 – one day

The wait for June, the month of my bilateral, is over. There is only one more day until my surgery. I'm ready. I want to get it over with. But then again, who am I kidding? I am nowhere near ready.

I want to be brave, but I am not brave. Why the hell do people tell cancer patients they are brave? We aren't brave, at least I know I'm not. No, what I am is afraid. I am afraid I will cry when I get to the hospital on surgery day and they ask me how I am doing. I am afraid of having no breasts. I am afraid of how I will look the first time I see my new reflection in the mirror. I am afraid the doctors will find more cancer in my lymph nodes. I am afraid of the pain I will have after surgery. I am afraid of the pathology report and what it might or might not say. I am afraid of chemo, hair loss and feeling sick. I am afraid of being treated differently by everyone. I am afraid of drainage tubes David must empty. I am afraid of scars and foreign implants. I am afraid David might see me as less desirable or not desirable at all. I am afraid of being weak. I am afraid of being a poor role model for my children. Mostly, I am afraid that my cancer has already spread, and I am dying. I am afraid of dying a slow, miserable death like Mother's.

I am afraid of moving forward into the unknown place where uncertainty waits. I am being pulled into a foggy, unfamiliar, yet way too familiar destination, and I do not want to go there. I am also afraid of standing still too long here in the present where cancer's tentacles are attempting to quietly take over my body cell by cell. No matter where I look there is fear. I must look forward because that is where hope, happiness, normalcy and life also glimmer along with the fear. I must move forward. I want to move forward, but I am still afraid.

Tonight David and I go to bed early. We lie together while listening to soothing music. It is the last time these two exact bodies will intertwine. It is the last time I will feel his hands on my breasts, and I try to file away the memory deep within me, but not so deep that I cannot find it again. He avoids touching them, already trying to disempower them. I wonder what he is thinking.

Like usual he falls asleep with no effort, but for some reason it doesn't bother me, in fact I am relieved.

"I'm sorry. I know I shouldn't be sleeping. I should be staying awake with you," he mumbles in my ear.

"It's alright," I whisper.

And it is. I am alone anyway. My mind, my thoughts, my fears belong only to me in the darkness. I watch the minutes slide by on the familiar clock that glows with a dim, yellow light. A text message comes in from Kay at 12:11 a.m. She, too, is awake and coping with a restless mind full of thoughts that seem to have nowhere to go, so they linger.

Finally, darkness and sleep are allowed to take over. The waiting is over.

-14-

More Decline

I stood outside my parents' bedroom door observing my father gently place his wife in bed as she moaned with pain. He lovingly adjusted her, tucked her in and kissed her good night. Oddly enough, in all my 50+ years, that was the first time I had ever seen my father kiss my mother. It took all my inner strength to maintain my composure while witnessing such an intimate moment. I now knew what true love and devotion looked like. I now knew what living out those vows until death do us part meant.

Minutes later I stood in front of the bathroom sink brushing my teeth while looking at my reflection in the three-way mirror and was startled by what I saw. I looked the same, yet I did not. I was a lot older, of course, than the girl who used to stand there brushing her teeth. I now looked like a daughter who had a mother with terminal cancer, tired and knowledgeable about unpleasant things.

I felt a connection to that bathroom where I used to spend so many hours getting ready for school and dates. When we moved into our green rambler on Central Avenue South, I was in sixth grade. My dad claimed the quarter bathroom off the kitchen for himself and Mark, relinquishing all claims to the main bath, except for the shower, knowing he was outnumbered by the females in his household. My mother, sisters and I were pretty successful most of the time sharing the bathroom space and the three-way mirror with its two adjustable sides we could maneuver into various positions for close up makeup applications and hair styling. Two of us could primp at the same time, one on each side mirror. The drawers used to overflow with makeup, curlers, hair brushes, combs and other various female things. Mother had everything in its place from the Kleenex box to the bottle of Jergens Original Scent lotion, to the wooden rack on the back wall holding towels in various shades of maroon, brown and beige. The wallpaper she so carefully chose and then years later wanted removed was still there, although it was peeling off in places. In an odd sort of way the bathroom was the room in which I felt the strongest connection to my past. It had a sense of order and familiarity to it.

But cancer had even intruded into the bathroom. The tub's glass shower doors had been removed and replaced with a shower curtain to make it easier for Mother, and in the middle of the tub was a white, plastic chair that looked ridiculously out of place, uncomfortable and intrusive. Mark had installed handlebars and a detachable shower head to further simplify the bathing routine. Even the toilet was transformed with a higher seat and handrails to make its use seem less impossible. Various cleansers and lotions sat on the counter along with pads, ointments and Fentanyl patches. For some reason we kept those patches in the bathroom instead of on the kitchen counter with the other meds. The free-standing, wooden towel rack had been moved so the wheelchair could get in, and the bathroom door was removed as well. We were no longer concerned with privacy. We just hung a sheet on a curtain rod in the doorway and hoped nobody came in at the wrong time.

Even the hook on the back wall of the bathroom was not as it should be. My mother's fuzzy, fleece, pink robe with sheep on it was supposed to be hanging there. It had been hanging there for years. She bought that robe uptown at the Fashion Lane when Madelia still had a clothing store, and it quickly became her favorite. She liked that robe so much she went back and bought three more for me and my sisters that year for Christmas. Mine was blue rather than pink, but it still had the sheep. We took pictures of all of us sitting on the sofa smiling in our new, fuzzy, fleece robes that were a strange match to the fuzzy perms we wore that year as well. Now other various robes and nightgowns that buttoned up in the front and were easier to put on hung on that hook.

I finished brushing my teeth feeling a little silly for feeling nostalgic about a bathroom, but then again it made perfect sense because my mother's presence was inside every nook and cranny of our used-to-be-green, now taupe-colored rambler, even in the bathroom.

In the morning it was quite a challenge for Mark to get Mother into the car, and then out again, into her wheelchair and on into the hospital for her appointment. Much patience was needed. Luckily, he had a lot of that. My dad mostly watched and held doors open, and I wondered what he was thinking. We were there for chemo, or rather, Mother was, but in a sense, we all were.

In January we had decided to try chemo, thinking perhaps we could slow down the cancer in Mother's liver. She was feeling so sick chemo couldn't possibly make her feel any worse, we had rationalized when Dad, Kay, Mark, Mother, her oncologist and I had sat huddled in the exam room contemplating what to do next. Mother was mostly silent at appointments now; Dad was too. It was up to their children to make the big decisions. We had decided to at least try to buy ourselves some time. That's what things had come to, bargaining for more time. Happy New Year to us.

We tried to not look back and second guess past decisions, like why we hadn't chosen chemo four years ago when this craziness all started. At that time we were told statistically chemo wouldn't increase Mother's survival odds much, if at all. That's really what doctors do, shuffle around statistics, make their best call and hope for a positive outcome. A lumpectomy and radiation were supposed to be enough. They weren't.

Despite our chemo efforts, Mother continued to decline. Her pain increased, so we increased pain meds. Her nausea increased and her appetite decreased. We were in some kind of terrible cycle, juggling medications, trying to find combinations that did not fight one another. She could no longer eat much and was losing weight fast. We still managed to get her to eat tiny meals of foods like mashed potatoes and scrambled eggs. They weren't meals actually; they were only bites of food. The little bits she managed to eat were only attempts to please us. The anti-nausea meds failed to be very effective.

I arrived again at my parents' house to go along for chemo session three. Kay and I took turns going to appointments. There were so many, we had to. Mark and Dad went to all of them. It seemed I was at my parents' house more than my own. My roles as wife and mother were becoming a blur in the background, part of a separate life. I arrived carrying two cases of chocolate-flavored Ensure. We were resorting to milkshakes for nourishment and added calories.

"I don't like the chocolate ones, I like vanilla," Mother informed me.

"I'll bring vanilla next time," I said.

She was clearly still annoyed and had no intention of drinking chocolate ones. She was rebelling in the only way she could.

Dad and I headed for the kitchen to try to figure out what we could convince her to eat instead.

"It's been an especially bad week," Dad said.

I already knew that from my phone calls. Still, she seemed happy to have me around, and for brief moments, I saw glimpses of the person she had been only weeks before

We arrived promptly at the hospital for round three of chemo and I took my seat beside Mother while hope was dripped into her veins. So much depended on that bag of mysterious, clear liquid hanging on a hook. None of us said much, especially Mother. We tried to act normal and make conversation, but the only normal thing happening was the snow falling outside our window. It looked lovely and peaceful, unlike the feelings of uneasiness and worry in my mind.

It felt strange to have a dozen or so patients sitting around together in one big room, all receiving chemo at the same time. We all pretended not to notice each other, but we all knew everyone was looking at everyone else wondering the same things. How sick did everyone else look? Who would beat the odds? Who was beginning chemo, and who was almost done? Who was wearing a wig, and who was wearing scarves and hats? Who was coping better than us?

Round three turned out very differently than the previous two.

After Mother and I got settled into our chairs, Mark and Dad left to go somewhere, I'm not sure where, just somewhere else. Almost immediately the first of many trips to the bathroom began. Each time, we dragged the IV-hook-on-wheels along with the wheelchair back and forth. Mother didn't want me to leave her side. I tried to keep my composure as nurses and I assisted her with too many bathroom trips to count. Only weeks earlier, I would have been embarrassed to be standing at my mother's side while she sat on the toilet. Now it was no big deal, and it felt reasonable and almost normal to carry around adult-size diapers in my purse. I was grateful to those nurses. Each time we called for them they responded cheerfully, always mindful of Mother's feelings and dignity. They were kind, caring and uncomplaining as they assisted her, and I thought about all they saw in that place day in and day out.

Finally, her doctor appeared to assess the bathroom developments. It didn't take long.

"Your mother is bleeding internally. We must admit her right away," he said.

Suddenly our already serious situation was even more serious. Our brief chemo campaign was over almost as quickly as it had begun.

There was more paperwork, more consulting and more phone calls to be made. We got Mother settled in her room and answered questions the nurses asked as they took her vitals. Dad, Mark and I wandered to another waiting room down the hall with large windows and no heat. Dad turned on a basketball game, and we sat and waited. We needed a little time to process the latest developments. A few minutes later we said hurried goodbyes to Mother and remarkably, her spirits were still quite good. We drove back to Madelia for another worrisome night with little sleep. Mandi and Radar seemed to know serious things were going on, as they greeted us more quietly than usual at the kitchen door.

The next morning when we returned to the hospital, the doctors had determined Mankato's hospital could not adequately deal with our serious developments. Mother must be moved to Mayo's Saint Marys Hospital in Rochester, Minnesota. There they would be better equipped. We knew none of this could be good, but Mother, Dad, Mark, Kay and I remained relatively calm. We were getting better at handling crises.

A doctor asked me to step into the hall for some private conversation.

"Do you understand the seriousness of your Mother's condition?" he asked. "She has already received several blood transfusions and may not survive the ambulance trip to Rochester. The bleeding has stopped but might start up again at any time."

He looked at me as if I were not understanding the magnitude of our latest crisis, but he was wrong. I understood all too well. I guess he thought I looked too calm or too together, but that was only on the outside.

On the inside my thoughts and feelings were jumbled and spinning. I was terrified by this new development but also hopeful new doctors at Mayo might be able to come up with some new miraculous strategy no one had thought of yet. After all, she was being sent to one of the best medical facilities in the world. She could not be in better hands. Surely they would be able to do something for her there.

Things were progressing too rapidly; there were too many doctors, too many decisions and too many questions without answers. I felt like I was running in some kind of marathon, struggling to catch my breath and keep up, but knowing full well it was a race I could never win.

Things moved even more rapidly after that. Nurses prepared Mother for her ambulance trip, and we exchanged unnaturally hurried kisses and goodbyes. Despite being so ill, Mother still did not like to rush her goodbyes, which in a different situation, would have been amusing.

Dad, Mark and Kay decided to go back to Madelia, pack their bags and head to Rochester that very night. I decided to wait until the next morning and headed back to Wisconsin, but all the way home I kept asking myself, what are you doing? Why are you not driving directly to Rochester tonight too? What if she doesn't survive the trip?

As soon as I got home, I informed David and Aaron that we would be making a trip to Rochester first thing in the morning. They asked few questions; they didn't need to as the worried look on my face told them everything.

It was another sleepless night of tossing and turning filled with thoughts of uncertainty sprinkled with flecks of hope. I no longer remembered what a good night's sleep felt like.

Elsie and Sophie did their best to comfort me with their gently wagging tails and understanding eyes. They were determined to stay by my side all night, and they did.

Thank God for my dogs, my secret keepers, I thought to myself as I finally drifted off to sleep dreaming about our much needed miracle and wondering what in the world we would do should we not get one.

-15-

No Miracle

There would be no miracle. Five days after she arrived at Mayo, Mother was discharged and sent home. How was it possible one of the world's most well-renowned medical facilities could just send us home with no solution? Where was our miracle?

The doctors had theories but never did find the exact source or reason for Mother's internal bleeding. After five days of hoping for our miracle, finally a young doctor gathered us together and attempted to explain our fragile situation. He chose his words carefully, drawing diagrams on a whiteboard hanging in Mother's room, attempting to make things more clear for us, but ultimately his message was simple and too clear; nothing more could be done. My mother was going to die—and soon.

The doctor seemed way too young to be so good at delivering such news, and I wondered how he felt coming to work each day, knowing he would have more bad news to deliver. How much good news did he need to give to outweigh the bad? I wondered if he went home at night, took off his white coat and forgot about cancer. Did he play with his healthy children and think his life would always be cancer free?

Mother didn't want to leave Mayo. She felt safe there, but we couldn't stay when there was no more to be done for her. That's not allowed. You can't just take up space in a busy hospital. So we packed up her things and drove home without our miracle. Her last days were upon us, and we all knew it.

So much for the New Year's optimism and hope, just like we flipped the calendar from January to February, we had to flip our mindset as well. Things had not turned out as we had hoped.

Betty and her daughter Jennifer arrived from Denver for a visit. Everyone knew it was a visit for sisterly goodbyes. They stayed at the motel in town instead of my parents' house because only our immediate family was allowed to see all of cancer's ugliness up close. We ate a chocolate ice cream birthday cake Betty bought for me and looked at slides of happier times trying to act normal.

Dad bought a slide camera years ago when my sisters and I were little, and he did a remarkable job of capturing those early years. Understandably, there was a lull in the number of slides taken after daughter number three arrived. The numbers picked up again after Mark was born. Over the years, my parents accumulated so many boxes of slides, they literally filled an entire closet.

Mother had always loved reminiscing and commenting about the various faces and places projected onto the wall or screen, but that day she looked at them silently without commenting or even interest.

Cancer continued to whittle away at my mother, stealing her away bit by bit. By that point, she spent all her time sitting or napping in her brown recliner. Our conversations became limited, often abrupt and always brief.

"Whatever you do, please do not say in my obituary I died after a courageous battle with cancer," she said out of the blue one night, giving me a clear directive on a matter obviously of great importance to her. "I do not want it to say that, I am not courageous."

"Okay." I assured her. "We won't say that."

Immediately I noticed the relief in her eyes.

Mother no longer slept in her own bed at night but rather used an in-home hospital bed Mark set up in my parents' bedroom. That hospital bed looked so out of place and intrusive crammed into the space between my parents' bed and Mother's closet, which we didn't need to get into much anymore since she only got dressed for doctor appointments. We told ourselves the hospital bed would make her more comfortable since it had buttons to push which would allow for sleep in any position. It would also give Dad more restful sleep, but we all knew what it really meant.

I fussed with Mother's hair using the big fork-shaped hair pick she kept in one of the bathroom drawers. I attempted to lift and separate what was left of her hair, which now looked and felt like matted netting. Only to please us, she tried on all the hats we had recently bought, and we all commented on how good she looked in them.

After Betty and Jennifer left, Susan and Michael arrived again for another visit. They would take over for a few days, but it was difficult to stay away. It was hard to not be selfish. It was hard to share those days with anyone, even my siblings. The bridge I was on for good now felt too crowded. It was supposed to be my bridge; I didn't want to share it.

I returned a few days later, and like usual Dad met me at the front door.

"Today is not a good day," he said.

He's never been a complainer, so I knew that was not a good sign, and I also knew he really meant Mother wasn't eating or drinking.

Mark had set up an impressive record keeping system in a black notebook, and he eagerly showed me the pages he had neatly divided into columns where we were to record what medications we gave, the date, the time and our initials so we wouldn't forget or screw up. The kitchen counter was lined with various bottles of Ativan, OxyContin, vitamins and Metamucil, the latter which we mixed with apple juice. Mother was obsessed with regularity for some strange reason even though she didn't eat anything so it seemed absurd to expect her bowels to work normally. Mark had declared the job of putting the Fentanyl patches on her every other day to be his job, as if none of the rest of us were capable, and maybe he was right. He wore rubber gloves when he tore a patch open and placed it on her stomach as if it was a major medical procedure.

Watching Mother become so lethargic made me question our extensive use of drugs. I was torn because I wanted her to be comfortable and not burdened with unbearable pain and nausea, but I longed for her real self. I felt robbed of the mother I once had, and I wanted her back.

At meal time, we wheeled Mother to the dining room table and tried coaxing her to eat teaspoons full of food, but it was difficult and we had little success. Dad stood nearby watching; he couldn't bring himself to feed her.

Trips to the bathroom were now mini-marathons requiring effort, patience and endurance—Mother's, plus that of two other people.

First, we coaxed and encouraged the simple act of rising up out of her chair into a standing position. That achievement alone felt like a monumental accomplishment. Next, we coddled and cheered each tiny step successfully taken with uncooperative feet and legs that felt heavy and unreliable. Then the strange-looking trio shuffled the short distance down the hall to the bathroom looking like some uncoordinated balancing act with too many clumsy participants. When the bathroom mission was accomplished, we slowly returned to the La-Z-Boy destination, prompting all the way like misfit cheerleaders. When finally seated again, we all sighed with relief, feeling exhausted and hoping the next trip was hours away.

Mother's last day at home began like most other recent days before it. After successfully getting her up out of the hospital bed, into the bathroom and dressed for the day, all of us were already worn out. The normal routine was for her to go directly to her recliner, but that morning my sisters and I decided to keep her in the wheelchair a little while longer. She needed to spend less time just sleeping in the recliner, we convinced ourselves. The next task was getting her medications down, but that did not go well. Mother had become extremely agitated and either could not or would not swallow her pills.

"Try again," I coaxed over and over.

She slowly took a pill with her shaky hand and stared at it as if concentration alone would get it to her tongue and down her throat. After several more unsuccessful attempts, she unexpectedly tossed the glass of water across the living room, startling us all.

"Is she angry we kept her in the wheelchair?" I asked Susan.

Susan shook her head in disbelief and had no answer. Such behavior was unsettling and disturbing because up to that point Mother had been cooperative and usually did what we asked. We were losing control over the few things left we thought we were still controlling. The day continued to deteriorate. Badly.

Luckily, the home care professional we had recently hired to check on things every few days arrived later that day and immediately saw the despair on our faces. She tended to Mother while Dad, my siblings and I huddled in the kitchen contemplating what to do next. We began to discuss nursing home options.

"I would like to try home hospice care," Susan said.

But Dad shook his head in uneasiness to that suggestion.

"I just don't think we can handle this anymore," he said. "It's just getting too hard."

I was torn between hospice and a care facility but felt the final decision was really his. He was her husband. Husband status trumps daughter status doesn't it?

Mother didn't seem able or willing to communicate and grew more and more agitated. I offered her a pen and paper to see if she wanted to tell us anything in writing, but all she managed to write were various, incomprehensible scribblings we could not decipher. Finally, after things went from bad to worse and after consulting with her doctor, the decision was made to hospitalize her.

Clearly, Mother was irritated with us and rightfully so. She didn't talk, appeared angry and glared at us a lot. Who could blame her? We had pretty much taken over her decision making, and I wondered if we really had the right to do that.

Once again, we prepared her for another painful trip out of the house. She grimaced as we helped her into her winter coat. She seemed to know she would not be returning home and motioned to have Mandi put on her lap.

"Goodbye, Mandi," she said. "You're a good little dog."

My mother spoke to Mandi but not to us.

Mark proceeded to carefully maneuver Mother in her wheelchair out the front door. I felt sorry for Mark having to take his mother away from her home for what was more than likely the very last time. What a painful and heavy emotional burden for an only son to bear.

-16-

My Bilateral

My alarm goes off at 4:10 a.m. with a loud, intrusive blare. The day of my surgery has arrived. The point of no return is here.

Surprisingly, I rise quickly out of bed and head for the bathroom to take the last hot shower I'll get for a while. I stand under the warm, soothing water and feel the steam build around me as it fills my nostrils. The steamy water cleanses my mind almost more than my body.

When I'm finished showering, I force myself to take one final look in the mirror at the familiar form. I need to take a final look. The reflection staring back looks the same as it did a few weeks ago before the madness struck. There are no signs of disease. No sense of urgency is apparent. I look the same. How is this possible?

I cannot look too long, however, because time is passing too quickly to allow me the luxury of slowness. We have to leave by 5:20. We are on a tight schedule. There is such precision to this cancer protocol shit. I dress quickly and finish packing, including far too many items I know I will never be using in the next two days. Still, I pack them. I pack my eyelash curler, my mascara, lipstick I never wear anyway (so why the heck am I packing it?), magazines, not one, but two books, my robe, slippers and even my curling iron for God's sake. I know I am kidding myself thinking I will want to put on any makeup tomorrow or the day after, but nonetheless I pack the stuff knowing full well it will probably all go unused. At least I'll be prepared for something.

Minutes later David and I pull out of the garage as it's getting light. When I return home in a couple days, I will not have my breasts. I will know more about my cancer and what I must do about it. I wish we could just keep driving anywhere other than where we are headed.

As we make the half-hour drive to the hospital, I spend the entire first half willing myself to not cry and hold it together, but I'm not sure I can manage. I'm not sure of anything except I am afraid. As if reading my mind, David takes my hand, and we continue on in silence. There is no need for either of us to say anything. There are no words for this stuff. But we are in this together. We always were. We always will be.

We pull into the hospital parking ramp at 6 a.m. sharp, right on time. We are so damn punctual. We appear to be so ready. Two other couples walk through the hospital entrance doors just ahead of us. The entrance is under construction, and we walk carefully amongst all the equipment and roped-off areas. I can't tell if it's the man or the woman in each couple who is having surgery on this day too. Both couples appear older, as if it's somehow more appropriate to have surgery at an older age. This should not be happening to us. The other two couples look us over carefully as well, probably trying to figure out which one of us is diseased, flawed or in need of repair. I wonder if it's obviously me.

It only takes minutes to get registered, escorted to the pre-op room, changed into a surgical gown and stretched out on the bed. Immediately, nurses and aides begin to hover, completing their assigned tasks. I sign consent forms without really reading them, answer questions and nod my head a lot. Everyone goes out of their way to be extra kind. Doctors eventually show up, ready to face another patient and another day of surgery as usual. My surgeon, Dr. Hower, appears looking calm and relaxed, and I wonder if there are doctors who do not have such a calm demeanor before surgery.

"Tell me, what are we doing today?" Dr. Hower asks.

He asks this while scratching his chin, as if I am here for a routine procedure or exam. I know the reason he asks this is because it's part of the checks and balances system before a surgery. I remember before Mother's lumpectomy her doctor asked if she was having a mastectomy. Umm, no, she was having a lumpectomy, we reminded him. Hence, I understand the need to confirm such things.

"Bilateral mas...," I start to say.

But I cannot finish saying the words. It's too hard to speak them out loud, and all of a sudden I am upset he would even ask me to do such a thing.

"Don't make me say it," I plead.

"Okay, I'm sorry," he says.

He pats my leg and says the words out loud for me. David and I just nod our heads to verify. It's all either of us is capable of doing.

The radiologist comes in next. I recognize him immediately as the same doctor who confirmed the mass the day of my ultrasound, but clearly he doesn't remember me.

"Oh yes, I remember you," I say.

I call him by his name, and he is clearly surprised and embarrassed by my better memory. Perhaps you should make little notes for yourself about each person you deliver bad news to so you can call her by name later and at least pretend to remember her, I want to say. But of course I cannot.

The third member of my team to introduce herself is my anesthesiologist. I am pleased to see a female face smiling down at me for a change. She smiles and smiles while she explains her role to me. I notice she has kind eyes framed with tiny crow's feet wrinkles that crinkle upward when she smiles, somehow making her seem even more kind and compassionate. Immediately I like her and feel calmer.

Next to arrive is the chaplain. It seems they have this whole process well rehearsed, like some surreal on-stage performance and each new "actor" knows exactly when to make his/her entrance.

"Would you like me to say a prayer for you?" the chaplain asks.

I say nothing.

"Yes, please," David says.

As the chaplain finishes his prayer, I glance at David and notice he is crying. The sight touches a place deep within me, and again I feel blessed to have someone who loves me so much. I realize just how afraid he is and has been too. I do not verbally acknowledge his tears, there is no need. It is one of the most intimate moments we have ever shared.

After the prayer session is wrapped up, David and I are instructed to say our goodbyes, and then I am whisked away down a long hallway to the operating room that feels like a refrigerator. I think back to the day of the mass sighting, remembering how cold the room I had my CT scan in felt. So much coldness.

"We keep it cold to help keep the bacteria level down," one of the three nurses I see explains.

While lying there flat on my back, I glance around the room and notice the three sets of bright, overhead lights, walls lined with glass cabinets and the operating table beneath those bright lights where I will be stretched out for the next six hours.

Then everything is blank.

-17-

Waking Up

Six hours later when I wake up in the recovery room, the first thing I notice is the large clock on the wall telling me it is a bit after 2 p.m. I'm surprised to find myself more mentally alert than I thought I would be, or at least I think I am. I hear nurses talking in hushed voices and watch them hovering nearby. I am relieved I have no pain, at least not yet. I feel like a spy peering out from my secret hiding place or an observer concealed under a fuzzy veil, quietly gathering information about someone else's life.

"He went for four lymph nodes," I incorrectly hear one of them say (it was actually fourteen).

Immediately I know they were not all clear. I can't hear many other details, the voices sound too distant and muffled, but I listen intently as if I am decoding safely guarded, classified secrets.

As I continue to wake up, I am acutely aware I have been lying in the same position for over six hours, and the idea of ever moving again feels like I might as well be trying to reach the moon. Eventually, after close to two hours, I am pronounced ready by whoever decides such things, to be moved to my hospital room where David, Peter and Aaron wait for me. Lindsay will come later tonight.

Still flat on my back, I am wheeled down numerous meandering hallways and finally end up in my assigned room. I brace myself when it's time for them to transfer me to my hospital bed.

"We'll count to three and then you try to lift your head," someone instructs.

I'm not sure if I am capable of blinking my eyelids much less lifting my head, but they count anyway, and I guess I do, because miraculously I am lifted via a blanket and placed into the hospital bed. Unfortunately, we must count and "lift off" once more for final adjustments in the bed. Finally someone else, certainly not me, determines I look comfortable enough and we all relax a bit.

Next I see David, Peter and Aaron standing over me with worried expressions on their faces. They continue looking down at me, as if waiting for me to say something profound.

"You look good," Peter says.

"Yes, you do," confirms Aaron.

I know they aren't telling the truth, but who cares? It must be hard to see your mother at such a moment.

Peter and Aaron leave almost right away so Peter will not be late for work at his summer job. Aaron will come back later with Lindsay, who decided to drive down from Fargo. I'm thankful for these three children who have become such capable, loving and caring young adults. When they were younger, I used to get sad thinking about them growing up too fast. Now I realize as adults our relationships are evolving into something even better. The best years are not necessarily those early ones. No one really tells you that when you become a parent.

Facing me must be hard for David, and I feel badly about this. He doesn't get to tell me all my lymph nodes were clear. That was supposed to be our secret code for things being okay when I woke up. If I heard the words "all clear," we could celebrate. If I heard the words "all clear," I would not need chemo. I don't get to hear them. We are both silent. Actually, I am too sick to think about much else anyway.

Coming out of anesthesia completely is like trying to free myself from quicksand. My mind feels clear and fairly alert, but my body seems stuck in slow motion, and I am unable to speed it up. Every movement I want to make from the simple task of turning in bed, to pushing the buttons on my remote, to the more monumental feat of actually sitting up and getting out of bed, feels mechanical, slow and difficult. When I do finally manage to sit upright in order to make my way to the bathroom, I move slowly, like a woman decades older, and I am overcome with nausea.

"It's okay," David says.

He gently rubs my back as I throw up into the long, narrow, plastic blue bag.

Eventually, I make my way to the bathroom accompanied by a nurse and attached to my pain-relief-drug-filled IV bag, which is in turn attached to a cart on wheels. The nurse has instructed me that I am allowed to push a button on the machine every so often for an extra dose. I push it. There hardly seems to be room for all three of us in the tiny bathroom with its annoying fluorescent light. Why do they always buzz? I glance at my pale reflection in the mirror, but I don't look for long. I don't want my gaze to make its way to my chest, not yet.

When you are recovering from surgery, you no longer take for granted simple bodily functions such as rising out of bed, putting one foot in front of the other, brushing your hair or teeth, emptying your bladder or even breathing. Such simple motions you normally do every day with little notice or appreciation now suddenly feel like the most valuable skills in the world.

Aaron returns this evening with Lindsay. I'm almost relieved Peter is at work and doesn't have to be here. We spend the evening just being together. I wonder what they are really thinking about, especially Lindsay. I remember thoughts I had while observing my mother struggle with breast cancer. They aren't thoughts I wanted her to have, at least not yet. It seems unbelievable I now have cancer too. However, I have just come through a successful bilateral mastectomy. My case will turn out differently. This is my new mantra.

The four of us sit around doing little, but accomplishing much, simply by spending time together. Later after they leave, I collapse into bed slowly; it is as much a mental collapse as a physical one. June 2 is over. Thank God. My bilateral mastectomy is done. I guess I am now officially a survivor. I have no idea what the hell this means. I do not feel like one. Regardless, for whatever reason this situation has been assigned to me, there is no turning back. I must look forward, just not tonight.

-18-

Watchdogs

People are remarkably adaptable, quickly adjusting to things they cannot change like cancer, nursing homes and even impending death. When forced to do so, a person's mind can adjust to almost any new situation. My newest adjustment involved having a mother in a nursing home who was dying from metastatic breast cancer.

The second time I walked through the dreaded doors of that facility while lugging a plant I had stopped to buy on my way, a bulletin board, my suitcase and other various necessities, it seemed a little easier than it had just days earlier. The place didn't seem quite so ominous and depressing. It even smelled better since the bags of urine-soaked linens that were piled up in the hall when I visited last time had been picked up. Thank God.

After being discharged first from Mayo and then later from the Madelia hospital as well, Dad and my siblings had successfully transferred Mother to her new and final residence. They had all been busy setting up her dorm-like room, and it looked quite homey and put together already. If there was one thing she had taught us, it was how to decorate. We put up pictures of all her grandchildren and great-grandchildren, as well as pictures of her favorite places such as the North Shore and the mountains. As if she would be residing there for months instead of days or weeks, we lugged in lamps, window decorations, snowmen, a CD player and CDs, numerous pillows, rugs, a calendar, a card table and chairs, puzzles, Easter lights and even a favorite Snow Village house because there was still snow on the ground after all. It looked truly impressive, that hodge-podge of winter and spring décor. Just as we were uncertain of which season to decorate for, we were unsure if we should be focusing on life or death. Of course, the real reason we busied ourselves with decorating her room so completely was because it was the only thing left we could control.

Everyone who entered her room commented on how nice and homey it looked.

"Oh, it looks so warm and inviting in here, I just love coming into your mother's room," one nurse in particular announced every time she appeared in the doorway.

"At least someone is glad to be here," I mumbled back each time.

I didn't feel like being friendly or making small talk. Not one bit.

Mother didn't complain or say much of anything, outwardly anyway. I wondered what she was really thinking, and I hoped she wasn't too disappointed in all of us for bringing her there. She no longer left her bed even to go to the bathroom. She seemed to have given into the inevitable. She didn't have much strength left for anything, only time and not much of that.

I assigned myself the new role of watchdog. I had little control over matters, it seemed, so I felt it was now my duty to watch out for Mother any way I could. I wanted to make sure she received good care in that new, unfamiliar place. I wanted to make sure the nurses and aides treated her kindly and gently when they turned her over or bathed her. I wanted to make sure the room was not too hot or too cold. I wanted to make sure the nurses came when we buzzed for them. I wanted to make sure they knew we were watching. Mostly, I wanted to be sure Mother was never alone.

"Is anybody going to stay with me?" Mother asked.

She spoke in almost an inaudible, child-like voice later that first night as we started putting on our jackets when getting ready to leave.

"I'll stay with you. I want to stay," I said.

Staying was as important for me as it was for her. Maybe more so.

"Oh thank you," she said.

Then she started to cry. She was so relieved to have someone volunteer to stay with her in that unfamiliar place. I was overwhelmed by her gratitude for such a simple thing.

Later that night, I stretched out as much as I was able in the green recliner that had buttons to push to make it easier for elderly patients to get in and out. I made futile attempts to sleep when Mother was restful. That night and the handful of others like it became like misfit sleepovers, minus the laughs. I looked forward to them, not the no sleep, but the incredible feeling of just being present. I was simply a daughter coming to realize the enormous privilege there was in help-ing her mother get ready to die. I had never felt more needed and appreciated, and it was hard to take turns and share the nights with my siblings. I started to bargain with God for more nights. I made promises in exchange for more nights. I was not ready to be mother-less. I needed more nights. Just more nights.

Usually Mother slept pretty well for a couple hours at a time at least. Two aides came in to turn her over every two hours or so, as they also did during the day. Some aides were very good at it, turning her over slowly and carefully, talking to her in kind voices while apologizing for the discomfort they knew they were causing. They arranged and rearranged the various pillows needed to prevent her from rolling back and ones between her knees to prevent bed sores. I learned quickly which aides and nurses were genuinely compassionate and which were in a hurry to get done and move on to the next pa-tient or task. In my new watchdog role I no longer kept quiet but boldly told them to slow down or be more gentle when it seemed they were too hurried or too rough. I sensed my presence annoyed some of them even though they pretended otherwise, but I didn't care. I was too worried, tired and stressed to worry about their feel-ings. A few looked way too young to work in such a place, and I wondered what they were doing there. What could they possibly know about illness and dying?

Each time after they left, I listened for the sound of Mother's breathing. If she didn't go right back to sleep, I sat by her bed offer-ing her sips of water through a straw, making small talk, holding her hand, rubbing her arm or just sitting there. Sometimes she liked to talk, and sometimes there was little or no conversation at all.

When it was my turn for night two of watchdog duty, I sat on my uncomfortable folding chair pulled up next to her bedside as close as I could get and let my eyes wander around the room. Sitting there in the semi-darkness, lit only by her Victorian-style Snow Village house on her nightstand and the pastel-colored Easter lights we strung along the ceiling with masking tape, I marveled at the almost ridiculous sereneness of the room. My tired eyes studied the familiar form lying in the bed. That face with its smattering of freckles, age spots and wrinkles looked so peaceful and untouched by illness while masked by the disguise of sleep. The sheets and blankets covered her frail body and the secrets of her disease. I closed my eyes and allowed memories tucked away and not recently thought about to drift into my mind like soothing, gentle breezes filtering in through an opened window.

Ironically, one of the earliest memories I have of my mother is of her lying in bed with me right there next to her. So long ago and such a different time. I was five and we were both taking an afternoon nap as she was expecting my soon-to-be-born little brother and undoubtedly was exhausted from being a mom to three active little girls.

Shortly after that day, my parents walked out of the house on a chilly Friday evening in early October and headed for the hospital where my brother would later be born. I watched them walk through the doorway that night feeling unsure about how my life was changing, but I knew it was.

At that time and all through elementary school, my family and I lived in a big old house on the north end of town that was cold and drafty in the winter and hot in the summer. On hot, humid summer nights my sisters and I sometimes slept downstairs, all of us sprawled out on the floor of the front porch which had a lot of windows we could open allowing summer breezes to cool us off, but usually we just waited for cooler nights to arrive. After stepping through the front porch entrance of that old house, you were in a large, open, parlor-like foyer. That room impressed me because of its size and for the fact that it really seemed to have no particular purpose and we had no furniture to put in it. The stairway leading up to the bedrooms was the focal point of that foyer and was my favorite place in the entire house.

Those stairs, though old and creaky, were quite impressive with their richly colored, polished banisters. Kay and I spent hours in that foyer and on those stairs turning them both into backdrops for whatever we conjured up or acted out. Once I ran into those stairs while crawling around on my hands and knees and gashed my face, nearly taking out my right eye and resulting in a dozen or so stitches. I've always been such a klutz. Those stairs literally left a permanent mark on me.

Upon leaving the foyer, one would find herself in the tiny living room where my family and I gathered to watch TV, which at the time delivered in black and white the entertainment one channel provided. We didn't mind our limited channel selection since we knew of nothing else, and each night seemed to bring a favorite show. Every Sunday night my sisters and I watched Lassie carry out her amazing good deeds no dog we knew could ever possibly accomplish, while we ate fried chicken and French fries Dad prepared. Saturday nights brought *Gunsmoke* and then *The Alfred Hitchcock Hour*, which somehow I often managed to be up late enough to watch until it became too frightening, and then I would be sent to bed. Once in a while we grew weary of our limited selections and attempted to tune in shows from another network. Some Sundays we tried without much success to watch *Bonanza* on NBC to see what that level-headed, knowing father Ben Cartwright and his three sons were up to on their ranch. Usually we became frustrated straining our eyes to see them on our snowy screen and resorted back to our limited, but clear-looking picture, on channel 12.

The basement of that old house was crumbling in places, and I was afraid to go down into that dark, damp place that seemed to hold mysterious secrets. Mother was a little afraid of that basement, too, so she always kept a table knife stuck into the door jam of the door that led down into the basement. I always wondered what kind of intruder a simple table knife could possibly keep out, but its presence in the door jam seemed to make her feel better, and that was good enough for me. You could also enter the basement from the backyard through one of those old-fashioned trap doors like the one Dorothy was too late to enter through when the tornado hit in *The Wizard of Oz*. That secret entrance made our basement seem even more mysterious, in my mind anyway.

Every fall, Mother began her mouse-proofing campaign in that old house by searching for nooks and crannies that might be potential entry ports for the unwelcome visitors. Any tiny opening was immediately stuffed with wads of steel wool. Despite her best efforts, a few of the tiny pests always seemed to find their way inside, causing her much angst when they scurried across the floor. I was secretly delighted by the reaction such tiny creatures caused.

When I was eleven, we moved into our newer and more modern ranch-style house on the exact same street, but on the opposite end of town. My parents purchased it from my piano teacher. Mother was thrilled on that chilly October day when we moved into our new home with its three bedrooms all on one level, shiny wood floors and picture-perfect yard. But mostly, I think she loved that new basement with its pine-paneled walls, real tiles on the floor and no crumbling walls with holes that needed mouse proofing.

Moving into that ranch-style house changed my life. Our new house was more modern with no bedrooms upstairs that turned into saunas on summer nights. Miraculously it seemed to me, our new house even had a window air-conditioning unit installed in a kitchen window and had more than one bathroom. Suddenly it seemed my family was living extravagantly. We now lived in a house with an attached garage and a real basement where we could entertain our friends, but the best thing about moving into our green rambler was that my piano lessons came to an end. I didn't mind the learning to play an instrument or the practicing, but I was frightened by my piano teacher. She was gruff, never in a good mood and impossible to please; I could never play quite to her satisfaction.

"Oh get up, here's how it should sound," she would abruptly say each week, clearly dissatisfied with my inferior playing. Then she shooed me out of the way and proceeded to play my assigned pieces properly herself.

I counted my blessings for many reasons the day we moved into our new home on Central Avenue South.

Unexpectedly, while sitting there next to Mother that night, voices jolted me out of my memories when two aides came into Mother's room to check on her and turn her over. They turned on buzzing fluorescent lights over her bed that felt intrusive and cold but necessary. Next they removed the blanket to turn her over, unveiling the stark reality of cancer, which included a catheter bag, pillows here and there holding her in place, swollen ankles and a delicate-looking, failing body.

When they were gone, Mother feebly asked for an orange Popsicle, so I buzzed the nurses' station and one appeared minutes later. Orange Popsicles were the only thing she could tolerate to eat, and I held it for her as she enjoyed the cold, soothing treat as it slowly melted in her mouth. She licked at it slowly and delicately taking in childlike amounts, reminding me of tiny birds Kay and I tried to rescue in the backyard years ago and attempted to keep alive with drops of water we gently squeezed into their mouths using droppers Mother gave us.

Days were disappearing too quickly, one sliding on into the next, and I wondered how many were left for us to all be together. Mother's good days were often followed by a bad day. Good days brought conversation, smiles and even laughter. She was able to keep water down, pain and nausea were under control and she enjoyed orange Popsicles. Such simple pleasures did not occur on bad days when nurses, aides, as well as family, could do nothing right. On bad days she could not even tolerate water. She scolded us, or worse, said nothing and listlessness took over. Blank stares grew longer and more frequent. We could give little comfort. On bad days, cancer and dying showcased their cruelest sides.

On day six, Mother's irritability grew especially quickly and even a visit with her pastor did not calm her; in fact, even he irritated her. She became belligerent as she told him a thing or two.

"You don't know what you are talking about," I overheard her say.

He continued to read from the Bible and tried to talk with her about heaven. She uttered obscenities at him. I had never heard my mother use such shocking language, much less when talking to her pastor. He merely shrugged off crude comments, obviously he had heard worse. He listened to her ramblings and calmly acknowledged her feelings. He gently reminded me it was the disease taking over, and I was grateful for his genuine kindness and compassion.

After he left that night, I called Kay to alert her about Mother's agitated state.

"Do you think you can come stay overnight too?" I asked. "I think it's going to take both of us to get through the night."

Kay soon arrived with suitcase in hand, and we started getting ready for bed. It was only 7:30, but that's when nursing home patients often get put to bed. The day had been too long, and we were all tired anyway, so it didn't even feel early. I settled into my recliner, pushing its various buttons attempting to find a comfortable position, and Kay left to go sleep on the sofa in the lounge area.

A few hours later, Mother woke up moaning, and nothing I said or did consoled her or made her more comfortable. She could not go back to sleep or lie still and didn't seem to know what to do with her hands. She nervously picked at her nightgown with the tiny yellow flowers on it I had recently bought for her. The blue pamphlet some-one had left earlier for us to read describing "behaviors to expect as death for your loved one draws near" listed this as one of those be-haviors to expect. She didn't respond to me when I tried to calm her; in fact, I just seemed to agitate her more. I became worried and called Kay on her cell phone. Seconds later she appeared looking a little un-raveled, and we both tried to settle Mother down. The situation quickly deteriorated.

"Help me, help me," Mother pleaded.

She kept on calling out the same words over and over again, softly at first and then more loudly and more desperately.

Ironically, we felt totally helpless. Nothing we did pleased or calmed her. It was almost as if she was another person, the mother I knew transformed into someone almost unrecognizable. She became more and more on edge and fidgety, as if something inside her was about to explode. Perhaps she was experiencing incredible pain. Maybe her body was attempting to put up one last struggle. Un-doubtedly, she was totally frustrated and angry with the world which was quickly becoming more and more useless to her. She was pissed off.

She glared at Kay and me. Our faces were inches from hers, and we struggled with what to say that might make some kind of differ-ence. I didn't recognize that person when I looked into her angry, almost scary-looking eyes.

"Get away. You know your breath makes me sick," she lashed out.

She yelled at us, calling us names I will never reveal in a piercing, hurtful voice I didn't recognize. She continued to curse at us and hurled insults our way as if we were strangers she didn't recognize about to torture her, instead of loving daughters she had never really raised her voice at before.

Kay and I looked at each other feeling bewildered, not sure what we should do or say next.

"How did we end up here like this?" I asked.

But there were no answers for anyone to give.

"Mother, nothing you can say or do will make us leave or stop loving you, so go ahead, say whatever you want to us. It's okay. Be angry. You have every right to be angry. Be damn angry. Yell. Scream. Swear. We can take it."

Kay and I kept repeating such words over and over, but they had little effect. That was the night we knew for sure this insurmountably wretched disease was taking over. It was devouring my mother's body with greedy and demanding swallows, no longer satisfied with slow, tiny nibbles. The mother we knew was disappearing before our eyes, and we felt helpless and afraid because we were powerless to stop it.

Her heart-wrenching wailing and pleas for help continued to grow louder, reaching a crescendo that frightened us. Surely they were heard throughout the entire wing of that place. I wondered what the other residents were thinking as they listened while lying in their beds. Did they feel empathy? Did they hear this kind of thing often? Or were they merely annoyed with us for interrupting their sleep? I imagined the desperate cries for help called out on a regular basis within those walls, some heard and some never noticed at all.

Finally, we frantically buzzed for the night nurses, surprised they hadn't already appeared on their own. Reluctantly, they arrived unsure of what they must deal with. Even though I knew they were not, they appeared judgmental, as if our room was now marked with a "scarlet letter" of hopelessness. They, too, tried to calm Mother but also failed. They glanced at Kay and me but said little. No words existed to comfort us anyway. Finally they succeeded in sedating her, but even medication took a long while to start working. It was an incredible, emotionally draining and difficult night with little sleep for any of us. I felt like all my energy had escaped through my pores. I had none left.

Miraculously, in the morning Mother remembered nothing about any of it.

"So, how did you sleep last night?" Kay asked.

We were both unsure of what Mother's response would be.

"Oh, I slept really well," she answered.

Kay and I looked at each other with tired eyes, feeling surprised but relieved for that small blessing. We even managed a small chuckle while we sipped our semi-hot coffee and decided no one else would need to know.

We were both watchdogs now.

-19-

Day After

After finally achieving my best two hours of sleep between 5 and 7 a.m., a new nurse beginning her shift comes in to check and record my vitals. I am pleased the night nurse has left for she was unimpressive to say the least. She completed her nursely duties adequately enough, but there was little caring, interest or genuine concern about my discomfort or needs. She yawned her way through her shift, clearly as unhappy to be in my presence as much as I was to be in hers whenever she came through the door. Oh well, she's gone. I didn't even bother to read her freaking name tag. She will remain nameless to me forever.

Mary is my new nurse, and she could not be more different. Thank God for nurses like Mary. She's petite, young and drop-dead gorgeous. She belongs in a movie or TV show. She has long, chestnut-colored hair, deep brown eyes and a flawless complexion. But this is not what makes her wonderful. The most striking thing about her is despite her youth and tiny frame, she exudes strength, compassion and competence. She is everything a good nurse is supposed to be and then some. Instantly I like her, and she at least pretends to like me. How can two nurses charged to taking care of me be so different?

After attempting to fix myself up in the bathroom with minimal success, I decide to order breakfast, not because I'm hungry but because I know I should eat something. After last night's nausea, I'll do anything to avoid that again if possible.

Minutes later my scrambled eggs, toast, fruit, juice and coffee arrive delivered on a tray by a cheerful young woman. Perkiness is overrated in a hospital.

I attempt a few bites, but of course, my timing's off as my surgeon, Dr. Hower, walks through the door, and my appetite immediately "walks out." He looks a bit nervous and I don't blame him. I know what's coming, more bad news. I wonder how many times he's delivered bad news already today or am I the first recipient?

"Unfortunately, your left sentinel node was not clear. You'll probably need chemo," he tells me.

I appreciate his bluntness. Still, he says this casually, as if it's no big deal. Almost on cue, my plastic surgeon enters next.

"My part of the operation was very successful," he says.

His words make it sound as if his part is not connected to the other part, and I guess in some ways it is not.

"Your tissue expanders are in, and I put in 200ccs already," he says. "So you will at least have some volume in each one right away."

It seems odd to talk about expanders and volume at this exact moment. I have cancer. I need chemo. I just had surgery. My body aches and feels foreign to me. Am I supposed to be grateful to have some volume already? Is this supposed to make me feel better? I know they both mean well, but they really have no clue.

Dr. Banich leaves quickly because even he knows cancer talk trumps plastic surgery talk today. I find it difficult to look Dr. Hower in the eyes. Suddenly tears start to cloud my vision. Immediately he gets fidgety and appears unsure of what to say. There are no words for this.

"I just need a good cry," I say. "It's how I process."

This gives him a chance to make an exit and I'm glad. I'm sure he's even more glad.

"You'll be fine," he says.

He pats my leg and leaves. I wonder how the hell he knows this because I sure don't. Doctors really should not say this. Why is this obvious to me but not to them?

I am no longer hungry. I sit in my uncomfortable, padded, blue-green chair that feels way too big and stare out the window at brick walls and parts of the hospital rooftop. The view stinks, but it would not matter if I were gazing at the Grand Canyon or Mt. Rushmore; all

I see is an uncertain future. All I can see is cancer and unclear lymph nodes.

I call David, feeling guilty since I was the one who insisted he go to work for a couple hours. I told him I would be fine. What was I thinking?

"I think maybe you should tell your mom, Steve and Lavonne not to come," I tell him.

I don't feel up to company, even if it's David's mother, sister and brother-in-law. I don't feel up to pretending to be strong when I am feeling weak and vulnerable. I don't feel like faking it.

"Okay," he says. "Whatever you want. I'll be right there."

Minutes later, I am fumbling for my phone and calling him back. It dawns on me that maybe he needs to see his family. Maybe he needs some support right now. I am a pitifully selfish wife, undeserving of such a caring husband.

"Let them come," I say, trying to sound confident and capable, knowing full well I am neither. "It'll do us all good."

I sense his relief and happiness. I have made the right decision. But panic sets in.

The first time people see you after your cancer diagnosis is awkward and somewhat difficult even for immediate family members. On top of that, throw in a bilateral mastectomy and the uncomfortableness factor rises a couple more notches.

When the time for their visit arrives a few hours later, I put on my fake façade of all-rightness and carefully reposition my sheets and blanket to conceal my chest. I wonder if it's obvious I've had two breasts removed within the last twenty-four hours.

It turns out to be a pleasant visit. We discuss Steve's past heart surgery as well as my surgery. Surgeries always bring out discussions about other surgeries.

"Nancy, you look really good considering the kind of surgery you just had," Lavonne says.

I guess this is a compliment. I merely smile and nod my head. I don't attempt much conversation. My presence alone is my participation today. I merely try to hold myself together and feel damn proud of myself for doing a decent job.

After an hour or so it's decided I am sufficiently tired out, and it's time to end our visit. David leaves with his family. He escorts them out to show them around, but we all know it's also to talk about me.

Let them say anything about me. I don't care. It doesn't matter what anyone says or thinks. I'm feeling incredibly stressed. And I'm in pain.

The nurse comes in and awkwardly takes my blood pressure on my ankle. She can't take it on either arm since I've just had numerous lymph nodes removed on both sides. She tells me it's really high, and she must report this to someone higher up. I'm exhausted both physically and mentally. I sleep.

The rest of the day I rest, wake up, visit with David and the kids and push the button on my pain-reliever-on-wheels that allows me more morphine every ten minutes. Lindsay's main duty is bathroom door monitor whenever I attempt to go. These attempts seem to take a really long time, and it's nice to have a female lookout. In the evening we fiddle with the TV remote and take a stroll down the hallway with me dragging my "drugs-on-wheels" machine. The short walk feels like a mini-marathon.

Eventually everyone is gone and I'm all alone. I'm worried about the night ahead and wonder how on earth I'll ever be able to sleep. Tonight there is a new nurse, Diane. She arrives with a small, round, white pill which will replace my IV drugs.

"Let's try just one," she says. "They're really strong, and you can always take another one later if one's not enough."

Stupidly, I agree to one.

Four hours later I awake to excruciating pain but somehow still manage to make my way to the bathroom and back. I am chilled and shaking. I buzz for the nurse. Diane reappears, takes my vitals, looks worried, consults with the doctor and hands me more pills. I knew one pill would be not be enough. Fuck this shit.

-20-

Discharged

David arrives early this morning appearing happy and eager to bring me home. I don't feel quite as eager. We sit sipping coffee as if we are staying at a posh hotel. We wait for Dr. Hower and Dr. Banich to arrive with further information and my discharge papers.

"Good news," Dr. Hower says. "I ended up taking out 14 lymph nodes and only one was positive for cancer."

I grimace inside at the thought of this supposedly being good news. What kind of good news is this? Our entire conversation seems insane, and I don't want to have it. I can only think about the here and now anyway. I can only concentrate on getting dressed and dragging my ass out of this hospital. I can only think about getting home. Yes, just today. Just get me through today. This seems like enough for me to take on, more than enough actually.

Dr. Banich's head, and then body, appear in the doorway, and he notices my drain tubes hanging loosely.

"You're leaking!" he says.

I laugh. Laughing feels good. When did I last laugh? His lame attempt at humor is just what I need. Good nurse Mary is back and helps me get dressed and organized. Then she wheels me out with David following close behind. He's brought Peter along too, who has gone to get the car. I am wheeled out into the world to face whatever is ahead. For now, just get me home. Just get me through today.

In less than one hour I am home, once again lying on my comfortable blue, leather sofa. I'm surrounded by a dozen or so pillows of various shapes, sizes, colors and firmnesses. Each one needs to be positioned just right, and it's no small feat to figure this out.

I love this old sofa. It feels like an oasis of sorts, right now the center of my life. It's the place where I rest, sleep, elevate my arms, watch TV, read, reflect, cry, plan, journal, feel sorry for myself, make phone calls, send text messages, worry, imagine worst-case scenarios, imagine best-case scenarios, sip on water from my hospital water mug, think and do nothing at all. I only leave it to go to the bathroom, eat and walk around periodically. It's merely a piece of furniture, but now it represents so much more. It's over ten years old. We purchased it the same year we took a family vacation to Disney World, in my other life. The life when there was no cancer yet for Mother or for me and when I had breasts that were mine. It's odd how someone can suddenly become emotionally attached to a piece of furniture, but then again, maybe it's not.

-21-

Orange Popsicles

"I just can't understand how she can keep going. She doesn't eat anything other than orange Popsicles," my dad said.

Those were the words my dad greeted me with upon my return to the nursing home. It was a greeting I received on a regular basis. Clearly he was mystified by it all.

Like many dying patients, Mother had begun the process of pulling away from us. That pulling away was difficult for the rest of us and only added to our feelings of helplessness. We kept trying to pull her back in. For a long time we kept trying to make her eat which was really just another attempt to keep her with us longer. Obviously, we knew when she stopped eating she wouldn't survive very long, so finally accepting the end of her food intake was very difficult. We had to let her stop eating. We had to start letting her go. Watching her completely stop eating and become weaker and weaker was one of the hardest things of all to watch. We all wondered how long she could survive on water and orange Popsicles.

Along with Mother's almost total end to eating, quiet thoughtfulness took over and a mysterious kind of listlessness set in. Conversation became less frequent; it was just too burdensome for her. It zapped what little energy she had left. However, an occasional burst of energy sometimes brought a smile, compliment, thank you or reprimand. We were always mindful of what we said because she was still very much listening to our conversations, at times interrupting with an unexpected comment or rebuke, proving she still had opinions to give and that she was still the wife and mother in charge. Sometimes she just said random things, blurting thoughts out that she apparently didn't want left unsaid.

"Nancy, you have been the most compassionate of all through this," she unexpectedly stated one day in front of all of us.

I wondered how such a statement made my dad and siblings feel, but probably what she really meant was I am most like her, able to show emotions more easily. In other words, I talk and cry more. Not surprisingly, nobody reacted to her comment anyway.

As the end drew near, Mother slept most of the time, and we were grateful for peaceful rest. Touch became her primary sense, and many moments were spent hand-holding and rubbing her arm which had a calming effect. She was sensitive to noise, movement and anything unnecessary. Her sense of sight had changed, or at least the appearance of her eyes, which seemed to be glassy and unseeing. The usefulness of her earthly body was ending; it was becoming heavy and cumbersome, held down by invisible weights. She had bouts of fidgeting and restlessness. She was ready to be done with this life's journey, and I felt torn because I knew she was ready to die, but I wanted our time to linger even if all we could do was be together in the same room. I knew that was selfish and wrong to wish for, but I was not ready like she was. Again, I bargained with God for more time, and made promises I could not keep. I just needed more time. I wanted more time. How would I know how to live my life without a mother in it? No one had prepared me for that.

We were all just waiting. We took turns sitting next to Mother's bed ready to jump up with a sip of water if she asked for one. We made small talk about the weather or Madelia's wrestling team which had members advancing to the state tournament. We looked at each other with tired, worried eyes, but mostly we just waited.

Sometimes while sitting there looking at Mother in silence, I wondered if what I saw would someday be my fate, too, and if my genes were filled with silent messengers of doom just waiting to deliver their secrets one day. There were even those fleeting moments when I sat watching her wondering why it was taking so long for her to die. I wished it could just be over. Such thoughts were quickly followed by thoughts of guilt and shame. What kind of daughter wishes her mother to die? Of course, what I was really wishing for was the end of her pain and suffering. She had suffered too much and for too long; it was time. She was ready. But cancer, the cruel beast that it is, wasn't quite done with her yet.

All we could do was keep being there, keep loving her and keep waiting. There was nothing else left to do.

-22-

Recovery

June 8

Today is Mother's birthday. I miss her so much. I wonder if she knows what's going on down here. If she does, she is miserable for me, but then again, there is no misery in heaven. Compassion then, she feels empathy and compassion and love. Lindsay calls me, remembering the day as well.

I'm feeling quite a bit better. I feel stronger and I'm eating well. I am able to read and journal without quite so much effort. I still find it unbelievable all this has happened to me. Why me? Why not my sisters? Such selfish thoughts, but still, why me?

"It's good this is happening now when you're young and strong," Peter tells me. "It's better than at a later age like Grandma."

I guess in some kind of twisted way, this is true. David tells me I am now cancer free, a survivor, or is this merely wishful thinking? No one knows for sure. Time will tell. I sure as hell don't feel like a survivor. I don't even know what that means other than I'm not dead yet I guess.

June 9

It's been one week since my surgery. Everyone says I've made a lot of progress. It's been a week since my last shower too. Sponge baths are adequate but not much more than that. Last night David washed my hair for me as I stood at the kitchen sink. I needed to wash my hair as I am going to my first post-op doctor appointment with Dr. Banich today. I can't go with greasy hair.

When his nurse removes the tape that was bound around my chest so tightly, it is the greatest feeling in the world. I was surprised by how little my incisions were "dressed." The stitches were only covered with a small amount of gauze, covered with Steri-Strips and then tightly encased with clear adhesive tape of some sort that was wrapped around my entire chest and back a couple times. The two incisions under my arms where the lymph nodes were removed were merely covered with Steri-Strips. When the tape is finally off, it feels as if I can breathe again.

Dr. Banich enters the room grinning, shakes my hand and says, "You're smiling today!"

"Yes, I'm actually glad to see you," I say.

And it's sort of true. But only sort of.

He examines me carefully with his eyes as I sit in the green dentist-like chair in the middle of the room. He wheels his chair around me with his eyes never leaving my chest.

"Everything looks really, really good," he says.

I wonder how a chest with two four-inch incisions where breasts used to be and two more incisions under my armpits, bruised, yellowish-looking skin and no nipples can possibly look really, really good, but he sounds convincing so I almost believe him.

I notice the two syringes filled with clear liquid. He picks them up and injects the mysterious substance into my new tissue expanders after first applying a small amount of numbing something or other. I feel nothing. I don't think I'll ever be feeling much in my chest again, or so I've been told. Suddenly, this realization makes me sad.

"I think I'll just do 30ccs today," Dr. Banich says. "We'll take it slowly at first. Your old breasts were probably about 450ccs."

"Oh."

What else is there to say?

Next, we leave the exam room and head into his office where he shows me pictures of other women with new breasts he has reconstructed. The photos only show the women's chests. You cannot see their faces. Of course, I know this is to protect their privacy, but it feels very awkward zeroing in on only their chests. Is this what really matters most about women, our chests? Sometimes I wonder. Sometimes I wonder what the hell I'm doing here.

Before we leave the clinic, we stop to pick up my pathology report. We will read that later, one thing at a time. David and I stop at the healing garden, a sanctuary of sorts, in the middle of this hospital. It's an enclosed atrium filled with plants, a water fountain and a player piano. There are benches and patio tables with chairs strategically positioned. We walk through the sunny space admiring the greenery, flowering plants, sound of cascading water and blue sky overhead. Whoever thought of putting something like this in a hospital was a genius. I'll be stopping here again. A woman dressed in gardening attire is busily planting deep pink geraniums, and she beams at me when I tell her how wonderful her work looks.

The day's outing was successful. I am still competent. I am still able to function in the outside world even without breasts. I am hopeful for the future, yet sad as well. I miss my old self. I miss my old breasts.

June 10

Today Kay, her husband Tim, and Dad are driving to Wisconsin for a visit. I have been looking forward to seeing them, but I'm glad they waited a week. I wonder if they were apprehensive while driving over here. I'm sure it's somewhat intimidating, even scary, to visit me right now. I suppose they wondered how I would look, feel and act.

They arrive carrying a box full of food that Kay has prepared. She is the prepared "doer" in the family after all. There are cookies, bars and cinnamon rolls, plus pumpkin bread from Tim's mother. Dad and Tim come into the house each carrying a hanging basket of flowers for the deck.

I stay seated in the middle of the blue, leather sofa surrounded by pillows with no intention of leaving my safe place. We talk about their three-hour drive, the weather and various other unimportant topics. You can't just jump into cancer talk too quickly. David comes home for lunch, and he and Tim leave to take a boat ride even though it looks like rain. At least they have an escape plan.

I open gifts from Kay and Susan, pajamas and a book from Kay and a candle and lotion from Susan. It must be hard for them having a sister who has breast cancer. They both know it could just as easily be them.

Peter and Aaron are home from work this afternoon, which is a good thing. They can keep Grandpa occupied with talk of college, baseball and summer jobs. I catch Dad looking at me with surveying eyes, but he says little directly to me. It must be hard to have had a wife and now have a daughter, too, with breast cancer. I wonder which is harder. I am the reminder of cancer, the reminder of unpleasantness, the reminder of loss. I don't like being the reminder.

Eventually Kay and I make our way into the living room for some serious woman-to-woman talk. I sit in the brown recliner trying to get comfortable.

"You can ask me anything you want," I say.

I am unsure about how little or how much she really wants to know, although I'm pretty sure she wants to know a lot since she might be contemplating a prophylactic mastectomy herself someday.

"How was it?" she asks.

So I describe my surgery, hospital stay, the pain, the IV, the nurses, my reaction to having no breasts, how my expanders feel, David's reaction, my drain tubes and how I feel right now. The words seem to pour out of me and I'm sure I'm sharing way too much, but I can't seem to stop myself.

"I'll show you my incisions if you want to see them, but I don't want to gross you out either, so it's up to you," I say.

I am feeling quite diplomatic.

"Yeah, I'll look at them," she says.

So we proceed to the bathroom, and I matter-of-factly start to lift up my white camisole tank top that has pockets for drain-tube paraphernalia sewed into it.

"Are you sure you want to see?" I ask one more time.

"Oh yes," she says.

I show her my four incisions and the drain tubes with surprisingly little hesitation or embarrassment.

"I don't even think it looks all that bad," I say.

Saying such a thing sounds rather ridiculous considering. Still, it's true. I imagined the sight to be far worse than it actually is. I'm sure she did too.

"No, it doesn't look that bad," she says.

Who knows what she is really thinking?

After a couple hours, the visit ends. It must be nice to leave my house and drive away from cancer. It must be nice to drive back to normal. I don't remember what normal feels like.

June 11

We head back to the plastic surgeon's office to remove the last of the drain tubes. It really hurts when he tries to gently twist and pull them out. I wince and cringe, but the brief seconds of pain are well worth it to be rid of the bastardly pieces of plastic. Good riddance!

June 12

David and I decide to take in a movie, but I can't make myself go into the theater. It's too soon. I can't do it. I'm not ready. Who knew this would be so fucking hard?

June 13

Today is Peter's birthday, and we celebrate by grilling hot dogs and eating a Dairy Queen cake. It's a simple but tasty birthday feast. Despite cancer, it's a good birthday.

This evening I start to worry about tomorrow's oncology appointment when the next phase of my treatment will be mapped out. I know my oncologist will recommend chemo, but I hold onto a thread of hope he may not. One fucking lymph node. I know I'm supposed to be grateful for that. It could've been worse. I am not grateful. I feel like I am being punished, but for what? It feels like another shoe is about to drop. Fuck cancer.

-23-

Chemo It Is

After checking in at our now familiar spot on the hospital's fifth floor, David and I find a place to sit and wait for my name to be called. I feel anxious and start fidgeting in my chair, but not for long because I am called back almost immediately.

After a bit more waiting back in the exam room, Dr. Nambudiri enters the room looking serious as usual. He is such a serious man, but then he has a serious job to do, plotting out treatment regimens for patients with cancer. I wonder what he does when he leaves work to forget about all of us. I wonder if he can forget.

He arrives with a chart in his hand. My data has been plugged in, and we begin to study bar graphs on his computer screen which indicate my expected fate ten years from now depending on what I do or do not do. If I choose to do nothing more following my surgery, my chances of being alive in ten years are 73.5 percent. If I add hormone therapy, I pick up 5.6 more percentage points. If I do chemotherapy and hormone therapy, I end up at an 86.8 percent chance of being alive ten years from this moment. Chemo allows me to pick up another 7.7 points. Such precise calculations and precise predictions now displayed before us in precise bar graphs allow me to see all the various scenarios. Who the hell figured all this shit out?

We discuss the various graphs and figures. We do the math. Just as I knew it would be, chemotherapy is recommended. This news is hard to hear. I feel sick. I feel trapped. Mostly, I feel afraid. And all this for seven or eight more points.

I stand up and start pacing around the room. I head straight for the Kleenex box because I know I am about to lose it. We start talking about the drugs that will be used.

"We will take the most aggressive treatment path," Dr. Nambudiri says.

This path sounds nasty and vile, but then this treatment course must kill cancer cells, so of course it must be even more nasty and vile than cancer cells. The words hang in the air again, just like they hung in the air on that other day not long ago. More words I want no part of.

"I'm way more afraid of chemo than surgery," I blurt out.

David and Dr. Nambudiri look surprised, almost shocked to hear this, but they say nothing.

"I'd rather have ten more surgeries than start chemo."

I decide I need to keep quiet. My words are not understood here in this moment by either of them. I attempt to calm myself, but I am unsuccessful and start to cry. I am crumbling again.

I cannot fall apart in this place. I will not. And somehow I don't, at least not completely. I collect myself, but I know it's a temporary collection.

"We'll need to put in a port," Dr. Nambudiri says.

He says this so nonchalantly, as if it's no big deal putting in a device that will be used to funnel poison more easily into my body. I feel sickened by the thought of needing such a thing and once again my tears appear.

"I'm sorry," he says.

Finally, it's time to leave the exam room and we stop at the desk to make still more appointments, or rather, David makes them because I am unable to do anything other than stand and walk. Again I vow not to lose it. I will not. I stand by the wall as it quite literally helps to hold me up while David looks at calendars and makes decisions about what day and time to begin my first infusion. Infusion, there's another despicable word. I stand there by the wall waiting, feeling as if I might explode. Or collapse.

An oncology nurse walks over to where I am standing and leans over to whisper in my ear.

"It's normal to feel overwhelmed. You'll get through it. You need courage and strength and you have both," she says. "Can I give you a hug?"

I don't want a hug. I want her to get away from me. I want to be left alone. I feel like screaming, but of course I cannot. I am not huggable, and I certainly do not feel as if I have one ounce of courage or strength. What bullshit. All I want is to get out of here. I want to retreat somewhere. I want to hide. I am not strong. I am not courageous. I am crumbling inside bit by bit.

I wonder why it's taking so long to make appointments. The receptionists glance my way sympathetically, one even winks at me. I must look a mess, but I suppose they're used to this look, the look of fear and helplessness. David is talking to my surgeon who has appeared from around the corner. I can't move, so I don't. They are talking, about me no doubt, but I don't care. My surgeon turns to me, holds out his hand for me to shake and asks me how I'm doing. I think to myself, why do you ask such a question? I just found out I'll be having chemo. How do you think I'm doing? He can tell by looking at me he will get no verbal answer. He doesn't need one anyway. We do shake hands and I attempt a smile. He says he understands, but he doesn't. No one does.

David and I drive home in silence. There is nothing to say anyway, not now. Once home I head for the blue, leather sofa and wrap my maroon-colored fleece blanket around myself. David sits across from me quietly waiting for the onslaught of tears he knows will be coming soon.

It doesn't take long. I am unable to keep them dammed up any longer and they flood out. I don't even try to stop them. I know my crying rampages worry David, so I get up and head for the solitude of our bedroom walls, comfortable white chair and view of the pine trees outside the window. I sit there and cry. I rock back and forth, sob louder and feel relieved to be able to stop pretending to be okay. I am not okay. I am miserable. I am afraid. I am angry. I feel cheated and unlucky. I am full of ugly feelings of disgust, despair, helplessness and self-pity. Yes, I feel sorry for myself and I don't care.

Chemo terrifies me. The thought of drugs with unimaginable side effects running through my veins makes me shudder. I don't want to feel nauseous, have diarrhea, get mouth sores or rashes, feel weak with no appetite, be tired all the time and lose all of my hair. Such thoughts and fears overtake my mind, and I am sickened by them. I am powerless to stop my tears, my feelings of despair and images of myself as bald from going through my mind. David doesn't even come to check on me. He wants to stay away. I don't blame him. I want to stay away from me. My mood is ugly. I am ugly.

Eventually, I find myself back in the family room lying on the blue, leather sofa where I allow the soft, worn cushions to surround me providing at least some comfort to my body, but not my mind. My expanders are hard and uncomfortable. My tears have slowed down but have not ended. They keep resurfacing. David seems unsure about what he should do, so he decides to go to the office and get some work done. I'm glad. I want to be alone.

I lose track of time, but I think three hours or so pass. I continue to rest, rotating between periods of crying and dozing. I am trying to process this latest punch, but this is the worst so far, and I am not doing a very good job. I would rather face ten more surgeries than chemo. Why doesn't anyone understand this? Surgery is easy. You have it and go home a day or two later. You recover. You look the same. You keep your hair. You do not vomit or run to the bathroom. You do not look sick. You do not look like you have cancer. People do not look at you with pity in their eyes. It does not last for months like chemo does. Chemo makes it all real.

I am vain, cowardly and full of self-pity, and I don't give a shit. I'm entitled this time. I think this might be the new worst day of my life. I will try to do better tomorrow but not today. Today sucks. I don't even answer phone calls. There is no one I want to talk to. I do not want to pretend. Cancer sucks. Chemo sucks.

I do talk briefly to Susan when she calls. I tell her I'm miserable and cannot talk any more. I tell her I want to feel miserable. I need to feel miserable.

"Of course you do," she says.

These are the best words conveyed to me today.

I cannot bring myself to leave the blue, leather sofa. I sleep here lately anyway, so it doesn't matter if I stay put. Before going to bed, David sits beside me and tries to make me feel better.

"We'll get through this. I will be here for you. I will support and help you however I can. We all will," he says.

"I know, but it still sucks," I say. "I'm angry. My expanders are uncomfortable, my body aches and I hate the idea of being bald and maybe sick for months. I will try to be stronger tomorrow but not tonight."

I can't seem to make him understand, and he leaves to go to bed. For once, I fall asleep almost immediately. I am physically and mentally worn out, and I'm pretty sure David is too. Adapting to all this cancer shit is exhausting for us both. And we know we are not done adapting yet, not even close.

-24-

Adapting

June 15

I feel a bit better today, so I guess I'm already processing and moving forward. What choice do I have?

June 16

I have three appointments today. I stopped keeping track of how many there have been. I know there are many yet to come. As David and I walk through the clinic's revolving doors again today, I think the people at the front information desk must be starting to recognize us. I know the receptionist on the fifth floor, the oncology floor, surely must. But maybe we all look the same to her.

Our first appointment is with my plastic surgeon. I am eager to see him because I'm worried about the swelling under my armpits. It doesn't feel normal. My left side feels like it has another breast growing out of it.

"Yes, things look really, really good," Dr. Banich says. "You actually don't have much swelling there."

His words sound reassuring. But I wonder how his pair of eyes can see things so differently than mine. Why do things feel so weird then? Come on, I tell myself. You just had a bilateral mastectomy. Of course things feel weird.

"Will these tissues expanders ever feel comfortable?" I ask.

"Not really," he says. "You will get more used to them, but they will always more or less feel like you have a bag of rocks on your chest."

No kidding. At least he is honest. I'll have the darn "rocks" until chemo is over, too, plus one more month after that. Implants have to wait now. Chemo takes priority.

"I think I can still get you pumped up to about 450cc before you start chemo," he says.

Today he injects 50cc into each side, so I now have 280cc. I'm over half way there. These strange, hard mounds on my chest are actually starting to be noticeable.

The purpose of my second appointment today is to have an echo-cardiogram, which was ordered by my oncologist to determine if my heart is healthy enough to withstand chemo. I almost hope it isn't. Maybe if they find an irregular heartbeat or something I will be deemed unfit for chemo. I wonder how often that actually happens.

The person to administer this test is yet another male; so many men have been peering at my chest, which now looks misshapen and odd. This technician's name is Jim. He's probably thinking, oh you poor woman.

"Don't breathe," he says every few minutes as he attempts to capture whatever it is he's trying to capture on that mysterious screen of his. He keeps apologizing for the discomfort he knows he's causing me.

"What exactly are you measuring or looking for?" I ask, trying to distract myself with conversation I don't really want to have.

"Oh, I'm measuring various things like the size of your heart's chambers, things like that," he says.

Next he moves the probe below my left breast and starts to press on the place my drain tube incision was, and I cannot bear the pain.

"That's not going to work," I say, wincing with discomfort.

"I'm so sorry," he says.

He continues on to the middle of my chest and then my neck. I notice I am now shaking, so I try to relax myself, but I can't. He continues to direct me about when to breathe and when not to.

Finally, I tell him he has to stop. No more. I can take no more. I'm not sure if he was even able to completely finish administering the test, but I don't care. I quickly get dressed so I can escape.

"If you ever need another one, it shouldn't be this bad," he says. "It's not supposed to be like a torture chamber."

Fuck you, I want to say, but of course I don't. I attempt a smile and head for the nearest exit.

"I know it's not your fault," I say instead.

The last appointment for this day which is starting to feel way overbooked is with my general surgeon, Dr. Hower, the one who removed my breasts, tumor and lymph nodes. I should hate him for carving me up, but I don't. In fact, I like him a lot.

He does a quick examination of my chest. It's the third time I've undressed today, and it's my chest's third examination.

"Things look great," he says. "You're healing nicely."

The three of us then talk about how chemo is the right thing to do. He acknowledges things probably seem overwhelming right now, and I want to hug him for saying so.

"Chemo months will pass quickly too," he says.

I don't believe that for a second. Next he pulls out what looks like a plug of some kind with a long cord attached to it.

"We need to put in one of these—your port. I would like to put it in the week before you start chemo," he says.

Hearing this freaks me out. We are supposed to be on our Bismarck, North Dakota, trip with Peter where he will do research at the capital for his master's thesis and then on our North Shore getaway the week before chemo starts. How can I possibly be on a vacation and have a freaking port in my body? I start to cry. It's all too much. I don't want to look like a chemo patient while on vacation. What kind of vacation would that be?

Dr. Hower feels very badly for me all of a sudden and decides to change the plan.

"We can do it the same day you begin chemo then," he says. "We won't spoil your vacation. That will work fine; July 13 will work fine."

"Thank you," I manage to say.

I cannot think about July 13, not today.

June 17

I decide I better stop feeling sorry for myself. There is much to be done before chemo starts. I must get off my ass, pull myself together and get on with things. It's hard, though, because my chest feels like it's in a vice grip, I'm still in pain and I'm terrified about chemo. I'm starting to think the women who opt out of reconstruction are the smart ones. I'd just like to have a calm chest. I don't even care about normal anymore, just calm would do nicely. And no pain.

June 18

David and I have been contemplating and planning for a few hours of intimacy tonight when he gets home. Surprisingly, perhaps, he seems genuinely excited about the prospect of having sex with me again. Lindsay is coming home tonight too, so we have to get an early start on things. Peter and Aaron are both at work. I spend a ridiculous amount of time deciding what to wear for this occasion. I rest often throughout the day preparing myself mentally as well as physically. I'm not sure what will really transpire. We've always had a healthy sexual relationship, most of the time anyway, so I'm pretty sure we'll be fine.

About 4 p.m. I decide to shower, get dressed, put on some makeup and a black lingerie top I can stuff into my jeans. My black high heels are the finishing touch. Then I take a pain pill and wait. As planned, David arrives home early around 5:30, and we head for the sofa in the living room where I arrange and rearrange pillows behind my back and try to get comfortable. Things proceed nicely, and after a few minutes we head for the bedroom. We move slowly and cumbrously at times, but we are successful in meeting our goal. We feel more committed, connected, loved and close than ever. I am grateful to have a husband who still sees me as sexy, desirable and whole. I am loved despite my imperfect body. I feel empowered, perhaps even beautiful, at least for a while. If he can love me without breasts, perhaps hair, eyelashes and eyebrows aren't that important either.

June 22

Attending a chemo education class is the highlight of today's activities, or perhaps more appropriately, the lowlight. It still feels unbelievable I need such a class. At first I thought it would be good for Peter and Aaron to attend as well, but then I changed my mind as they didn't seem interested. Besides, why put them through it? They'll be educated enough in a few weeks. Plus, they remember Grandma.

My kids know way too much about cancer already.

Nurse Candy, our chemo class leader, escorts our small group back into a secluded conference room. She's a middle-aged, blond woman wearing a two-piece, green uniform who appears to be someone used to being in charge. David and I take our seats around the large table in the center of the room, and she hands me a folder of information. It's immediately obvious she already knows which one of us is the patient. Another couple sits across from us, again decidedly older than us, and I once again think I'm too young for this shit. This woman has obviously undergone a mastectomy too. The only other patient is an angry-looking, pot-bellied man wearing a red t-shirt and glasses. He sits down while keeping his arms folded firmly across his chest, clearly unhappy to be here. He is accompanied by his wife and two younger women—perhaps daughters, and a younger man—perhaps a son or son-in-law.

After introducing herself and welcoming us to a class no one wants to be at, Nurse Candy shows us a video about the side effects of chemotherapy. I sit watching actors pretending they have cancer and listening as the narrator spews out what seems like an insurmountable list of possible negative side effects to be prepared for. Suddenly I wonder if the benefit is worth it. I despise the idea of funneling poison into my body and killing healthy cells as well as cancer cells. What if I don't even have any cancer cells left? But then, what if I do? There are no absolutes here other than I will lose my hair, be tired and look and feel like hell.

I become perturbed with Nurse Candy when she announces to the entire group, in what seems to me a cavalier attitude, what I can expect from my chemo drugs.

"Nancy, you will most definitely be losing all your hair."

You are invading my privacy. What right do you have to say these things in front of strangers? I want to ask, but I keep quiet. I mean, is there really anyone on the planet who doesn't realize hair loss is a common side effect of chemo? I want to leap out of my chair and strangle her but remaining still and silent seems far wiser as she may very well be the nurse administering my chemo one day soon. I don't want her to think I am some nut case.

"Oh, I am well aware of that," is what I do manage to say.

I sit there pretending losing my hair is totally expected and will be no big deal. Why do I feel a need to pretend? Cancer patients should not have to fake it, or hide their true feelings. It's not fair to have cancer, and it's certainly not fair to feel you must smile your way through any of this shit. I hate the unspoken expectations out there that make having cancer even harder.

The grand finale to our class is being taken on a tour where we are paraded toward the chemo room and allowed to peer into the mysterious space. I realize one day soon I'll be the one being peered at through the glass. At the conclusion of our tour, David and I head straight for the elevator, eager to escape the secrets of the fifth floor for another day. We don't want to know any more.

Our next stop is the local bookstore where I nonchalantly meander through the rows until making my way to the health and disease section where I search for books about chemo.

"Are you finding what you want?" a sales clerk asks.

"Oh yes," I lie.

I am feeling embarrassed and maybe even a little ashamed, although why I have no idea. There aren't many books about chemo on the shelf, but I manage to find one that looks informative and hopefully helpful appropriately titled, *The Chemotherapy Survival Guide*. Well, that sounds like the book I need alright. I scan the cover and table of contents and then hand it over to David so he can buy it. I don't want to face the cashier. Reading it will be bad enough, I don't need to purchase it. Why does having cancer suddenly feel like something to be ashamed of? I can't even bring myself to walk up to the counter and buy the freaking book

Our last stop for today's excursion is the mall where we decide to be extravagant and go see a movie in the middle of the afternoon. I feel ready to sit through a movie. Not that many people are free to go to a movie on a Tuesday afternoon, so of course, the theater is unnaturally empty and quiet. The movie we have chosen is *Get Him to the Greek*, and as expected, it is mediocre with vulgar humor, drug use scenes, raunchy innuendoes and no shortage of nudity and bare breasts. Oddly enough, we enjoy it anyway, maybe even because of the outlandishness of it all. We munch on popcorn and sip our Sprite enjoying each other's company as if we are on a date. My mind keeps wandering back to reality throughout, but at times five or even ten minutes go by before I am reminded of cancer, having no breasts and chemo.

June 23

Today I am getting behind the wheel and driving myself to an appointment for the first time. It's time for another expansion, and I am going by myself. This is allowed if I am not taking too many pain pills. I'm not, at least not today before the expansion. I feel like a teenager being given the car keys and allowed to drive alone for the first time. It feels good to be out on my own again.

I arrive at my appointment right on time and sit waiting for my name to be called. I observe the other patients waiting, easily picking out the ones obviously on chemo. I can't help but wonder what I will look like when I sit being observed by others like I am doing today. How sickly will I look?

"Let's go for 80ccs today," Dr. Banich says.

"Okay," I agree. "Why not?"

That was not a smart decision.

I walk through the parking lot a few minutes later realizing I just made a big mistake. The newly added weight from this increased volume immediately starts tugging at my right side. It feels like I have a brick attached to my chest, and I have intermittent stabs of pain. Despite my discomfort, I foolishly decide to stop at the mall as planned to pick up some shoes I had chosen an earlier day. I walk in slow motion and make attempts at shopping, but it's impossible to turn to look at things, much less bend over to try on shoes, so I slowly make my way back to the car. I need to get home. Shopping was a mistake. 80ccs was a mistake. Maybe reconstruction was a mistake. I can barely get into my car. All the way home I pray no one will run into me. I don't think I could survive an airbag hitting my chest. When I pull into my driveway, I'm so relieved. Home never looked so good.

Dr. Banich, you bastard, I mutter to myself. Life used to be simple and pain free, didn't it?

-25-

Last Goodbyes

Time was now a most elusive thing. I wanted more and gratefully welcomed each hour and day that arrived, uncertain of how many were left for Mother. On the one hand, time passed slowly, minutes silently blending into hours, as we sat and waited for the outcome we did not want to see unfold. On the other hand, I felt powerless, unable to slow time's momentum as each day too quickly rolled on into the next. What happens to time that leaves us?

Regardless, time was running out and staying away was becoming impossible. When Peter came home for spring break, I felt the immediate urge to get him to the nursing home to see Grandma again. So Peter, Aaron and I headed back to Minnesota for a visit. I wasn't sure how to prepare them, especially Peter who had not seen his grandma since Christmas. It turned out I didn't do a very good job. I prepared him mostly for personality changes and not the physical ones. The unbearable night Kay and I recently experienced was fresh in my mind, and I was afraid Grandma might say something mean to Peter on what could be his last visit with her, so I tried to prepare him for that. I didn't want his last memory of her to be an insult or unkind comment. It didn't matter what she said to me, ugly words that had no meaning could not harm me. A few ugly words could not erase all the good ones.

When Peter walked into her room, I realized I had been wrong. I should have prepared him more for the physical changes because the changes since Christmas were dramatic. I had grown accustomed to them since they had evolved slowly, however, they caught Peter off guard.

My mother's appearance was indeed much altered. She had little hair left and wore a turban. I felt badly about the hair. She only received three rounds of chemo which turned out to be pointless anyway. If we had not bothered with chemo, she could have kept her hair. But actually the turbans were quite becoming, providing her with some much needed color. Kay picked out two, one pink and one turquoise. Mother had always felt she looked best in pink, so that one was her favorite. Her complexion had almost a waxen look and was quite yellow due to her failing liver function. She looked small and weak lying in her bed propped by various pillows, her petite frame appearing even more vulnerable and fragile. Her cheekbones were sunken since she had probably lost 30 pounds. Her teeth were not in good shape as they had become difficult to get brushed properly. But, the most striking change was in her eyes. When you looked into them, death was staring back. There was no luster and they, too, were yellow. They seemed glazed over, and sometimes when she looked at me, it felt like she was not seeing me at all.

Peter stepped into her room, took one look and burst into tears. Seeing my six-foot son crying over his grandma broke my heart. He turned around and left in order to collect himself. In a few minutes he returned and proceeded to sit by her bedside and hold her hand.

The sight was quite sweet because Grandma was very coherent and actually almost glad to see Peter crying. I heard her tell him how much that meant to her. She liked to see people showing their emotions so openly. It made her feel better somehow to see someone's feelings unrestrained and just allowed to spill out. Not that the non-criers cared less. She just appreciated seeing feelings openly expressed, at least that day she did.

Thankfully, it turned out to be one of Mother's good days. She and Peter engaged in special conversation carried on through tears. Ironically, she ended up comforting him. Aaron sat close by, talked and cried with them too. I listened and watched, feeling proud of my boys but sad, too, as they witnessed dying close up. Such memories will always be special ones for them, and I was grateful to be observing such moments.

Later Lindsay and Josh arrived from North Dakota and they, too, shared special moments with Grandma. I was thankful Lindsay now had Josh in her life to help her get through such a thing and that all my children were able to spend precious moments with their grandma so close to the end and say goodbye.

We all walked around Mother's room quietly, talking mostly in whispers. I felt unable to breathe deeply or think clear thoughts. Death was coming for my mother soon. I could feel its unwelcome presence right there with us in the room.

Tuesday arrived and I returned to the nursing home after spending a night back home in Wisconsin. The nursing home was becoming a more familiar place now, not quite so harsh and cold. Had it really only been two weeks since we checked into this place? There was no sense of time now; what good did it do to keep track of time anyway?

I was drifting along waiting to step off the bridge I never wanted to be on. I tried to look back at my old life before the bridge, but it was becoming distant and foggy. I wanted to go back to that life, the life with my mother always in it, but I knew I could not. Looking ahead to the other side seemed impossible.

Susan and Michael arrived again from Tennessee, so I prepared to leave, allowing them to have some time alone with Mother. I think she had been waiting for them. Once again, I put my face close to hers and whispered goodbyes in her ear.

"I'll be back on Thursday," I whispered. "Wait for me."

-26-

Cranial Prosthesis

Today is an important day in my personal cancer shitstorm. It is the day I will buy a wig, or a "cranial prosthesis," as the insurance company prefers to call it. Such a term sounds outlandish and over the top, but regardless of what we call it, I will be needing one soon. This day symbolizes something very concrete, my acceptance, though forced, of my new reality. Within a month, probably less, I will lose all my hair, not just the hair on my head, that is not cruel enough. No, I have been told I can also expect to lose my eyebrows, eyelashes, pubic hair and all the hair on my arms and legs. Hair loss is one of the most cruel blows cancer and chemo deliver, and I am not prepared. How does a woman prepare to be bald? How does one get ready for that?

David and I drive back to Woodbury where we started the narrowing down process of wig selection a couple weeks ago. Thank goodness we got an early jump on things. Today we will get down to the nitty gritty and make our final selections. Today is also a sultry July day. Heat and humidity hang thick in the air surely churning up storms for later tonight. It seems ironic; this is so not a wig-wearing kind of day.

We enter the Merle Norman store this second time feeling at least somewhat more at ease. We are relieved to see Cindy, the same sales clerk, is working again. Today we are faster and we waste little time.

We are on a mission and head straight for the vanity area while Cindy retrieves the wigs we managed to select at our previous narrowing down visit. The three of us study, analyze and finally choose the two we think look most like me even though none of them really do. Our first selection is a rich-colored brown, bob-style wig, and it actually looks pretty good. Cindy trims the long, side-swept bangs precisely so they will fall below my brow line, in case my brows should disappear. We make our second selection, deciding to order it in two other colors as the store sample one is not the right shade for my complexion, though how we know this for sure I do not know.

David and I leave the store carrying out our newly purchased Rene of Paris wig, wig stand, wig brush and specially formulated wig shampoo. The Parisian sounding brand name sounds lovely, even glamorous, but there is no glamour in losing all the hair on your body because you have cancer and will be having chemo. Still, we leave the store feeling better than when we came in. We have successfully hobbled over another hurdle in this shitstorm.

We head home hoping to make it before the Mother Nature sort of storm arrives.

-27-

Getaway

It's time to head to my plastic surgeon's office for yet another fill up. I have determined I will allow him to inject only 30ccs in my tissue expanders today. I want no discomfort, or at least as little as possible. David and I have our pre-chemo getaway planned. We will leave at noon. Time will stand still, or at least slow down, for one weekend.

We are proud of ourselves for leaving right on schedule. It will be our last pre-chemo opportunity to be a normal couple uninhibited by the drugs that will soon be flowing through my veins causing God knows what kinds of side effects. I'm glad I do not have the port yet. I was smart to make a fuss over that.

We enjoy the leisurely three-hour drive to Duluth, and then we continue on another thirty miles more to the lodge we have chosen. After some confusion about our proper room assignment, we finally settle into our honeymoon suite on the second floor overlooking the lake. We laugh about how we are taking up a honeymoon suite since we've been married for over three decades. It's ironic because there's a wedding taking place here tomorrow, and we wonder if there is another honeymoon suite available. Maybe they wanted this one. Too bad, we deserve it more.

There is something about Lake Superior that has a calming effect on my soul. Maybe it's the name itself, Superior; this lake is exactly that. Maybe it's the vastness of the open body of water which constantly changes, much like my mood. Sometimes it's calm and still, looking like a mirror. Other times gentle ripples endlessly chase each other. And sometimes gigantic waves crash onto the rocky shoreline, as if boldly and noisily claiming superiority of water over land. Or maybe the appeal of this place is in the trees and rugged cliffs that butt up to the shore creating picturesque scenes perfectly suited for post cards. Perhaps it's the clear, crisp air that feels unspoiled and worth breathing in more slowly and deeply. Beauty and serenity exist in this place. I hope people don't screw it up.

We spend time sitting on our balcony, sipping champagne, eating quiet meals, watching the water, reading and enjoying each other's company. On Saturday afternoon we observe the wedding ceremony from our balcony vantage point. The bride, groom and all their guests don't bother to look up even once, so they have no clue they have two more uninvited wedding guests. They all look hot, nervous and relieved when it's over.

Night comes too quickly and I don't want to sleep because then morning will come and we must leave this place. Next week brings with it reality, cancer and chemo. I want to stay here and hide from it all. The wedding guests congregate on the deck below our room becoming noisy and distracting. Finally, we are forced to close our windows in order to sleep. People are spoiling the serenity already.

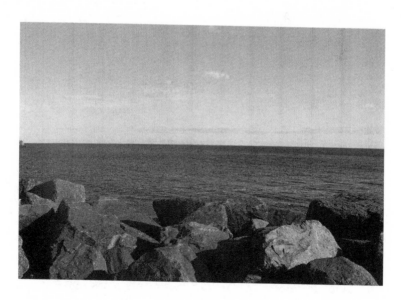

Lake Superior

-28-

Four Simple Words

"We just lost her."

Those were the four simple words Kay used when she called to tell me the news. I had been expecting such news for a while, but hearing the words said out loud caught me off guard. How could four simple words instantly change my life forever? Despite the fact I had been preparing myself to hear them for months, I wasn't yet ready to hear them. It wasn't supposed to happen that day, perhaps the next day or the day after that, but not that day. I wasn't ready to step off the bridge. I wasn't ready to be on the other side.

When the call came, I was getting started on the three-hour drive to visit Mother, a drive that had become so routine-like over the past few months I hardly had to think about it. I mindlessly merged onto I-94 and headed west joining the seemingly endless stream of cars, as if we were all being pulled along by some magnetic force somewhere up ahead. Like all interstates, I-94 is one more impersonal ribbon of cement connecting drivers to their destinations more quickly, by-passing cities and towns that will only slow them down. When you stop at the strategically placed rest stops, travelers mind their own business avoiding eye contact as if that, too, would only slow every-one down.

The drive to Madelia had become so familiar. I knew exactly what time of day to leave to avoid Twin Cities traffic. I knew how long it would take to reach familiar checkpoints along the way such as the

St. Croix River that provides a natural boundary between two states, The Lindbergh International Airport and the intersection where I always switched onto U.S. Highway 169 South. I knew the most convenient places to stop for gas or a bite to eat. I could almost pinpoint the exact time I would pull into my parents' driveway. It had become a soothing drive, a transition time between my life in Wisconsin and my caregiving life in Minnesota. Those three hours belonged only to me, and I looked forward to solitude and anonymity on the highway.

On that day Peter was along. He was still home for spring break and we were hoping to have another "last" visit with Grandma, so how could it be that we had just lost her? Such untimely and unwelcome news did not fit into our plan. Kay's words sounded vague, as if Mother was lost in a crowd, and we could just go find her.

I didn't have to say anything to Peter. He heard my conversation with Kay, realized he would not be visiting his grandma that day and immediately started crying.

I continued driving, staying surprisingly calm, almost as if our plans for the day remained unaltered. I didn't stop, pull over or even cry right away. I clung to that steering wheel.

The day was sunny and warm for early March, and suddenly it annoyed me that the sun's rays continued to feel so pleasant and inviting as they streamed through the car windows. What a stark contrast to my mind which was quickly becoming cloudy and confused, filling up with thoughts of disbelief, uncertainty and an overwhelming sense of emptiness. It seemed I could actually feel Mother's earthly presence leave me, a very real physical sensation of being cut off from a part of my life I would never be able to return to. I knew at that moment I was a changed person forever. There was no going back to my old life in which I had a mother. I had to step off the bridge for good. I was on the other side.

I also felt left out. My sisters were both there at the end and I was not. Why couldn't Mother wait for me too? Why did she feel like she could go ahead and die without me?

I was envious of Susan and Kay. They were able to watch Dad hold Mother's hand as she slipped away. That memory is theirs forever, and I did not get to share it. My face was not one of the loving faces Mother saw in her last moments. Was she looking for mine? Did she wonder where I was? Did she ask for me? Such thoughts were pointless and selfish, but I couldn't stop them from entering my mind. I hoped they knew how lucky they were to be there. Mark had not been there either, and I wondered how he felt. In a cruel twist of irony, I had gone back to Wisconsin for my annual physical. As my doctor and I sat discussing my next mammogram, my mother was soon to take her last breath. Cancer is fucking cruel.

"Mom, do you want me to drive?" Peter asked.

"No," I said.

I was still unwilling to give up the security of that steering wheel. I was in shock or just not ready to fall apart yet. I'm not sure which. I was forced to stay focused if I kept driving.

Peter and I didn't know what to do next. We didn't know if we should keep going or turn around and go home. We felt confused and indecisive. We decided to keep going. Eventually, I pulled over after Peter called David, Lindsay and Aaron with the news. Peter had cried and now it was my turn.

-29-

Three Hours Later

Peter and I arrived in Madelia exactly three hours later, right on schedule. We called Kay again and she, Susan and Dad were all back at the house already. Mother's body had been collected, so there was no reason to continue on to the nursing home. We went directly to my parents' house.

Once again, I felt left out. Couldn't they have waited? What was the rush? Did the nursing home need the bed emptied so quickly?

I had missed out by not seeing Mother in the place where she had taken her last breath. Somehow that seemed important, and I had missed that chance. I wondered why no one thought of this. I should have told them to wait for me. Missing any small detail of this life-changing event seemed wrong. I couldn't miss anything else. I felt an overwhelming need to store up every detail in my memory because such details were all I had left and I needed them all.

When I walked through the backdoor entrance into the kitchen of my parents' house for the first time as a motherless daughter, everything seemed eerily strange. Mandi wasn't even barking like usual to greet me. Instead she stood there quietly, waiting patiently for me to bend down and pat her on the head.

I was amazed at the calmness of my siblings. Susan stood at the kitchen sink doing dishes, a perfectly reasonable thing to be doing. But all I could think was, how can you possibly be washing dishes at a time like this?

Kay was standing nearby in the middle of the kitchen with her arms folded, as if we were gathering for one of our family celebrations like someone's birthday or Thanksgiving. Mark had arrived from Mankato and was in the living room feverishly vacuuming, as if having a matted down carpet with crumbs mattered.

When my siblings saw me, they didn't stop what they were doing or say anything. I'm not sure what I expected. Maybe I wanted them to rush over and hug me. Maybe I wanted to see them crying inconsolably. I guess they didn't know what to say or do, so they waited to see what I would do. I was amazed they all appeared so calm and secretly disappointed they didn't look more upset, even though I knew they were. I wanted everyone to look as miserable as I felt. I wanted their pain to look as obvious as mine felt.

I proceeded directly to my dad, hugged him and immediately broke down crying. I must have appeared pretty unraveled because everyone just looked at me uncomfortably. Dad patted my arm and tried to comfort me the best he could. It had always been hard for him to show emotions. He was never a hugger. He was an arm patter. I always knew he loved me even though he never said to me the words, I love you.

Mother always rationalized Dad didn't express emotions easily because he was raised in a strict German family where he was taught one's emotions were best kept unrevealed. His parents did not believe in open displays of affection. I think his mother was pretty strict, and I often wondered what his childhood had been like. Of course, he didn't talk much about it.

Dad and his family lived in Kulm, North Dakota, a small, rural community south of Jamestown. When my grandfather was a small child, he and his family had immigrated to the United States from Russia looking for more opportunity, but mostly to avoid service in the Russian army for the children. Somehow they ended up in Kulm, North Dakota. Kulm's claim to fame was the Hollywood TV and movie star Angie Dickinson once lived there. I was unimpressed since I had never heard of her at that time, but Dad was quite proud of this fact. I even mentioned it once to some of my friends hoping to make some kind of impression, but they were even less impressed than I had been. Years later I would sometimes see Angie Dickinson in her own ABC TV show, *Policewoman*, and I wondered if she had any recollection of Kulm, North Dakota.

Dad had three older brothers, two older sisters and still has one younger brother. He graduated from Kulm's high school early at age 16 and left for college, looking for opportunity beyond Kulm. It seems as if residents of small towns are always in a hurry to leave.

We visited the house Dad grew up in infrequently, but I was fascinated by it. My favorite place in the entire house was the stairway. I was drawn to those stairs because they had no carpet, unlike stairs in other houses I knew. Instead, they were painted a shiny, light brown and felt slippery underfoot. I was intrigued by their steepness and how they seemed to rise straight up leading to large bedrooms that felt unfamiliar and in need of exploration.

A house next door was home to a witch, or so my sisters and I believed. The witch was old and cranky and didn't like noisy visiting children. Sometimes she came out of her house and scraped the sidewalk with her rake yelling at us to keep out of her yard and garden. My sisters and I were deathly afraid of her but at the same time mesmerized. The thought of her coming out of her house terrified us, but tantalized us, too, and we secretly hoped she would appear. Dad said she was harmless and "not quite right upstairs" and that we should ignore her, but that explanation only made us more intrigued. She was just old and crotchety, but to us she was a witch.

I was never close with my paternal grandparents. My grandmother died when I was only four, leaving me with few memories of her. One I do have is of when I barged in on her accidentally while she was preparing for bed and brushing her long, gray hair that she always kept in a bun at the base of her neck. I had intruded on a personal ritual, and I felt badly about that.

I always felt awkward around my grandfather. I might have even been a little afraid of him, probably because he looked so old and gruff with his gray hair, bushy eyebrows and mustache. His voice and laugh were raspy, and he coughed a lot no doubt due to heavy smoking. In addition to that smell of cigarettes, he teased me a lot and did tricks like making a penny disappear and then miraculously making it reappear behind his ear. He didn't visit us often, but when he did it was usually around the World Series time. He loved baseball and sat for hours in his car listening to games. That always seemed odd to me, but now I understand Mother probably just didn't want him smoking in the house.

"It's okay," Dad said.

Such simple words of comfort offered, as I stood next to him crying while he awkwardly patted my arm.

But no, I thought. It's not. How can you say that? It's never going to be okay again.

At least he looked sad, confused and lost as he stood in the middle of the living room appearing unsure of what he should do next. Somehow seeing him looking so vulnerable made me feel better. My siblings all looked way too busy putting things away.

I didn't want to start putting Mother's things away; it felt like we were putting her away. I wanted to keep everything just as she had left it if only for a little while longer. I wanted to touch things she so recently had used, like her water glass, tube of red lipstick, bottle of perfume and box of Kleenex. I wanted to feel her presence by touching such personal items. I wanted to sit in her chair and feel how its shape had conformed to hers and smell the pillows that surrounded her frail body just weeks ago.

I wanted to shout at them to stop. Instead, I said nothing. I guess some of that old German heritage had been ingrained in me as well, and I just stood there silently, feeling alone and out of place, unable to force words out of my mouth. It felt as if something was being drained out of me. I felt upset, maybe even a little angry with my siblings, as they continued putting Mother's things away.

Of course they were only trying to cope in their own ways too; there was a lot to do after all. Still, I couldn't help feeling resentful and disgusted with myself for feeling so powerless to say what I wanted. Why couldn't I just ask them to stop or at least slow down? Instead I felt immobilized, unable to say or do much of anything. My mind and my mouth were disconnected and uncooperative. I was being washed away; someone had pushed me off my bridge. I did not want to get off yet. I was drowning, unable to swim to either side to save myself. I was lost.

Finally, I sat down next to Susan to ask what had happened that day and to find out why she hadn't called earlier. I knew I shouldn't ask why she hadn't called; that would probably only make her feel badly, but at that moment I didn't care. Perhaps I even wanted her to feel a little guilty; she got to be there and I did not.

"Mother didn't look right today," Susan explained.

She hadn't looked right for quite some time. We both knew that.

"We thought it was going to be just another day. Mother did seem quieter this morning when we came into her room. Her eyes appeared glassier, and she didn't even blink much. I don't think she even knew we were there; she just slipped away while we were sitting around her bed," Susan continued.

But you were there, I kept thinking. Did she realize how incredibly lucky she was? I kept such selfish thoughts to myself. I was not a good sister in those moments.

As everyone continued to clean up and put things away, I began to feel agitated and started pacing around the house. I needed to see for myself that Mother was really gone, so I found Peter and we decided to drive to the funeral home. I needed to see Mother. I had the feeling everyone except Peter thought this was a bad idea, but I didn't care. I was feeling very determined.

When Peter and I arrived at the funeral home, we rang the doorbell and knocked and knocked, but there was no answer. We tried the back entrance. Again, no answer. We were too late. Why was I always too late? Everything was locked up and no one was around. Again I wondered, what was everyone's hurry? Why did things have to be put in order so quickly? Everything was moving too fast for me.

We got back in the car and drove home on familiar streets I'd been on a million times. We met Dad, Susan and Michael at the corner on Main Street. They were headed for the grocery store, again doing something that seemed incredibly absurd, but of course, it also made perfect sense. We had to eat.

As I glanced up and down Main Street, the storefronts stood waiting like familiar friends from my past ready to once more welcome me through their doors. Some of them had been transformed into new businesses with updated signs and storefronts, trying to cover up the facades of the '60s and '70s, and some were still remarkably unchanged.

The dime store where my friends and I walked through cluttered aisles countless times after school while the store owner suspiciously watched our every move with his twitchy eyes was now a quaint bakery/coffee shop. In that space where we once stared at a candy counter filled with countless sugary delights, you could now instead gaze at pastries and smell freshly brewed coffee.

The movie theater where I saw pretty much every movie that came to town still looked exactly the same. Sometimes my friends and I managed to sneak into "R" rated movies in that theater. IDs were not often checked, and everyone knew who we were anyway. Such behavior seemed bold and daring to us. That old theater with its lighted marquee made our main street seem more substantial and city-like. Our small town with its thriving movie theater had more substance than similar, neighboring small towns we frequently visited which had none. Everyone in town took pride in that movie theater.

I thought about all the times I walked up and down Main Street with my friends on warm summer nights talking and laughing as we pretended not to notice boys driving by too fast in cars. We spent hours leisurely strolling back and forth on those tree-lined sidewalks. There wasn't much else to do. We were never afraid or worried about much back then, and I certainly never once thought about walking home to a house without my mother being there. She was always there waiting for me, no matter how old I became. And now she was gone.

When Peter and I got back to my parents' house, it felt forever changed, as if the house itself knew something important was missing. It felt empty and quiet. How could it look exactly the same but yet feel so totally different? I thought about how Mother would never again walk through the familiar rooms, rush to the front door to greet me or stand in the doorway waving goodbye to me when I left.

I sat down in Mother's brown recliner, wrapping the blanket that still hung on the back around my shoulders. I closed my eyes and took in the smell of her perfume that still lingered. I felt many emotions, but mostly I felt lost, disconnected and alone. Nothing I had felt or experienced before compared to how I felt at that moment. I sat in her chair feeling emotionally paralyzed, a daughter suddenly totally uncertain about how to carry on without her mother.

-30-

Arrangements

I didn't have to sit around wondering what to do next for long. When someone dies, there's plenty to get done. Maybe this is a good thing because it keeps you preoccupied with death's busywork. Two tasks that felt undoable loomed, going to the nursing home to clean out Mother's things and planning a funeral.

Mark, Susan and I drove one last time to the nursing home. When I walked through the doors, I realized in two short weeks I had become accustomed to the place that so recently seemed foreboding and unwelcoming. Since our loved one had died, we were now outsiders, no longer belonging in such a place. Mother's stuff had to go to make room for the next insider. Staff members and residents tried to hide their uncomfortable gazes as they glanced in our direction, unsure of what they should say or do. Why doesn't anyone ever want to deal with death?

When we entered Mother's room, we saw her bed covered in a white sheet with a single red rose and a card saying, *In loving memory of Jual Schuldheisz.* It took my breath away. It looked lovely, a kind gesture carried out by some unknown staff member. I was deeply touched by that simple act of kindness and respect.

We proceeded to un-decorate the room. We didn't talk much, there was no need, and we didn't feel like it anyway. In a trance-like fogginess we began putting away Mother's things. It felt eerily strange knowing she would no longer see or use any of them. I repacked her rose-colored suitcase with the nightgowns I had recently bought along with other miscellaneous stuff like her glasses, lipstick, makeup, brush, mirror and slippers. I heard her voice telling me to take care of her special hand mirror. The frame was made of ivory and it really was quite valuable, although its real value was of the sentimental kind because it had belonged to her mother. Such personal items were silent secret keepers, containing bits and pieces of information about the person who had so recently used them. Examining Mother's belongings a stranger would quickly learn about her favorite fragrance, lipstick color and her petite size.

We carried all the CDs, rugs, pillows, pictures, calendars, lamps and other miscellaneous decorations we had carried in only days before back to the car. It didn't take long and soon the day's first task was finished.

Planning a funeral was next.

At that point, I had been involved with the planning of four other funerals. My first experience was after my cousin, Robert, was killed in an accident. He was nineteen. People aren't supposed to die when they are nineteen. Francie, Robert's mother, had been in Minnesota for Mark's high school graduation and that same night Robert's pickup careened into a deep, poorly marked hole in the country road he was driving on back in North Dakota. He was killed instantly, they told us.

I always wonder about that statement officials so often make intending to comfort family members. If your loved one dies instantly, is that supposed to make you feel better? I know they mean well and of course, there is comfort in knowing your loved one did not suffer for minutes or hours, but it seems to somehow minimize their death experience, like it somehow wasn't that bad. How can a living person judge that?

I got the call about Robert's accident the morning after Mark's graduation as I was getting ready to go to work. I don't remember who called to tell me, Mother, or perhaps, Susan. Mark's graduation celebration was forever tarnished by tragedy. Despite the devastating news, I went to work that morning thinking I had to be there to finish my end-of-the-year duties in my second grade classroom. What an idiot I was.

That same day, David had the most excruciating job of all, picking up Francie from her hotel room in the Twin Cities where she had been staying. Later he described the unimaginable screams and wailing he heard as he approached her room unsure of what he would find when he opened the door. He also accompanied Francie on the flight back to North Dakota and had the heart-wrenching task of collecting Robert's personal effects, as well as picking out a suit for Robert's brother Gary to wear to the funeral. No one else in the family was emotionally capable to do those tasks; we were all reeling from shock and unable to do much of anything.

When I arrived in North Dakota a day or so later, I sat down next to Francie on Grandma's sofa and looked into her eyes red from crying, struggling to find words to say. What do you say to a mother whose teenage son has just died?

"How are you doing?" I asked.

I was ashamed of my inadequate words. Francie managed a weak, welcoming smile.

"Better now that you are here," she said.

She was comforting me that day; no comfort existed for her.

Somehow we managed to make the necessary arrangements for Robert's funeral. We buried Robert on Memorial Day weekend.

Three months later we were gathered again to plan another funeral in North Dakota. My grandfather had died after a lengthy illness from bladder cancer. We buried him on Labor Day. We started and ended that summer with funerals.

Chester Hurtt was a stout, pot-bellied man with a quick temper but an amazingly kind heart. He had an infectious laugh that captured the attention of everyone in the room and often those in the next room too. Sometimes when we were eating in a restaurant and he let out one of his famous laughs, I felt embarrassed as I watched heads turn to look at our table. Such a loud, boisterous display made the shy, young girl I was uncomfortable. As I grew older, I learned to love that infectious laugh, along with the embellished stories that often preceded it. I came to realize people were actually drawn to him partly because of that laugh, his wonderful story telling ability and overall zest for life.

My grandpa spent his entire life doing what he loved most, farming in North Dakota. His greatest joy was working in and showing off his grain or potato fields to anyone he could convince to go along with him to admire them. Every summer my siblings and I spent hours driving around the countryside looking at his fields, of course, he did most of the looking. Often he would stop the car right in the middle of the road, pull off into the ditch and drive straight into a field, all the while jostling around his grandchildren who, of course, wore no seatbelts. Our eyes would pop open wide as we marveled at the sounds of rocks and overgrown grass scraping underneath his vehicle. Such rides took place not in a pickup but rather in whatever large, totally impractical sedan he was driving at the time, such as a Lincoln Town Car or Buick Electra. All that scraping and bouncing made us feel quite wild and adventurous. We knew our parents, but especially Grandma, would not approve of such shenanigans, so we and Grandpa kept our wild-ride secrets to ourselves.

Grandpa farmed fields all over the county, and showing them all off to us was quite time consuming. At times we grew bored with the seemingly endless fields that all looked the same to us, but we never let on. We knew any complaints would be unkind and insensitive, and besides there was almost always a treat at the local Dairy Queen when our touring was complete. When my sisters and I were old enough to see over the steering wheel, Grandpa would often let one of us drive, though of course we had no license or permit, much less any actual driving skills.

"What if we get pulled over?" I asked him more than once.

"Oh don't you worry about that, I'll take care of everything," he said every time.

And we knew he would. We felt wild and free driving around on those North Dakota backroads with Grandpa, no matter which one of us was behind the wheel.

We all knew Grandpa's death had been accelerated by Robert's. Robert was supposed to take over the farming, and that could no longer happen. Grandpa's dreams had been shattered by cancer but even more so by Robert's death.

A couple years later we planned Grandma's funeral. No one loved and stood up for her grandchildren like Grandma Clara did. Not only did she never say anything bad ever about any of us, she didn't allow anyone else to either, at least not in her presence. Just like Grandpa, Grandma was never the same after Robert's death. Shortly after both their deaths, she suffered a stroke from which she never recovered. I still miss her.

We planned my father-in-law's funeral in March of 1993. Helmer Oliver Stordahl was a kind, hardworking family man of Norwegian ancestry. Years earlier, he had suffered a heart attack and surprised everyone by not dying, but rather living another twenty years. We all knew those additional years were bonus years. He lived to be 88 years old, so there was a whole different feeling to the planning of his funeral. It was still hard, of course, but knowing he had led a long and full life with no apparent suffering from illness at the end brought a more peaceful feeling of acceptance for his loved ones. Relatives gathered at his house and sat around fondly telling stories and jokes about him. It was a comforting way to celebrate his life and say goodbye.

The next funeral to plan was my mother's.

Funeral homes, especially older ones in small towns like the one in Madelia, are such uncomfortable places. As soon as you walk through the doors, you can feel the unnaturalness of the surroundings. Once inside, you feel the emptiness even though operators try hard to make things feel homey. Maybe they try too hard. You can't escape that cold, empty feeling. They must crank up the heat just before mourners arrive. Often there is that old Victorian-style furniture placed close to the walls leaving vast spaces in the middle for mourners to mill around in, and of course, the Kleenex boxes are always within easy reach. The environment and entire experience of being there just feels totally weird.

The funeral director who assisted us in the planning of Mother's funeral was kind and caring, speaking to us in a soft, understanding voice, offering his condolences sympathetically, and I wondered if he used the same words for all grieving families. Or did he have a script for each type of death scenario? He carried a clipboard with a list we went through robotically, as if checking off a list at the grocery store. He marked off our selections for memorial card handouts, urns and thank you cards, and I thought how odd it was to sum up someone's life in three or four paragraphs on a 4 x 5 memorial card.

Next, we had to pick out a plot and order flowers. For those two tasks we split our group up. The men headed to the cemetery, and the women headed to the florist shop. Before leaving the funeral home, I decided to ask the director if Mother's body was still there, not yet cremated.

"Yes," he said.

"I would like to see her," I said.

His nervous reaction immediately indicated he did not think this was a good idea. But I didn't care what he thought.

"It's already been a day. But of course, I will get her ready for you if you insist, but you will have to come back later," he said.

I did insist.

"I'll be back," I said.

I noticed Susan and Kay exchange worried glances.

"I don't think that would be a good memory of Mother for you to have," Kay said.

"No, I don't think so either," Susan agreed.

I wondered why they thought that. What were they so worried about? Of course, they were just trying to spare me more pain. They were clearly uncomfortable. They kept looking at each other while shaking their heads, but that only made me more determined. They didn't understand. They were with Mother when she died; they knew she was really gone. I needed to see for myself. I needed to say good-bye. I would definitely be back.

We left the funeral home and headed to the florist shop which was filled with fresh spring plants and blooming flowers; it felt warm and alive in that shop. I breathed in the aroma of life permeating the air which was in stark contrast to the funeral-home smells of damp-ness and death.

When we finished, I returned alone to the funeral home wonder-ing if I had given the director enough time to get Mother ready. What did he need to do? I had no idea. When I arrived, he still seemed nervous and concerned about how I might react.

I spent just a few minutes with my mother one last time. Yes, she looked different, and I wondered how someone could be here one minute and gone the next. Could death really just be the end of it all, or were those lessons I learned as a child about souls and heaven true? I was surprisingly composed while looking at Mother for those few moments. I told her one more time what a great mother she had been. I told her I loved her. I adjusted her necklace, a simple cross on a silver chain she had asked me to buy for her when she was sick.

After a few minutes, the funeral director stepped up to my side indicating my time should be up and apologetically informed me I would have to remove that necklace; jewelry wasn't allowed in the cremation process.

I bent over and kissed my mother goodbye for the very last time. I thought about the many goodbyes we'd exchanged through the years knowing there would be no more. I noticed how cold she felt. She had no hair and wore no turban, but to me she was beautiful.

Insisting on seeing my mother one more time was a good decision. I am forever grateful for getting that last chance to see her. It was important to say goodbye. I needed to say goodbye.

-31-

A Funeral

Mother's funeral was on an early day in March. It was a spring-like day, the kind that teases you into believing winter might be over soon, but of course, you know better. It was a day of warm sunshine and puddles everywhere from melting snow, yet the wind still had a cold, biting chill.

I spent the better part of an hour staring into my closet wondering what to wear to my mother's funeral. What kind of attire is appropriate for a daughter to wear to her mother's funeral? Finally, I decided on black pants and a beige blazer that will now always be remembered as the outfit I wore to Mother's funeral.

When we arrived in Madelia, we checked into the local motel. It felt odd staying in a motel in the town where my parents' house was. Mother would not be happy if she knew we were staying at a motel. However, we had decided earlier it would be easier and less crowded if we weren't all at Dad's trying to get ready in one bathroom.

We spent the funeral eve gathered together at the house with Dad. I decided Susan definitely still is the real cook of the family. Once again she put together a complete meal with three courses even though none of us cared much about eating. We spent most of the evening scavenging through old photos, searching for just the right images to represent the timeline of Mother's life for display on the memory board we intended to have at the church. How do you summarize a person's life with a dozen or so old photos?

On the morning of the funeral we left for church too early, but there wasn't much point in waiting around longer at the house or motel. Baskets overflowing with beautiful flowers were placed at the front of the sanctuary. Mother's urn was positioned among the flowers looking smaller than I expected. I guess a person's ashes don't require a very large container.

Months earlier Mother had told me about her somewhat surprising decision to be cremated. Lutherans don't typically go that route, at least not ones from her generation. Two of her best friends were a minister and his wife, and the three of them apparently had thoroughly discussed this topic. Since she had their approval along with Dad's, that was good enough for her.

The church had changed since I went there as a girl. An addition had been added, enlarging the social area, the space you need for feeding people after weddings and funerals. The church women, some of my mother's best friends, were bustling in the kitchen getting the noon luncheon of sandwiches and various assortments of cake ready. I wondered how it felt to work at a funeral for one of your friends.

We stood around awkwardly waiting for people to come through the doors to give their condolences. When mourners finally arrived, they said kind things or tried. I can't remember much about what they said. Some faces I recognized. Some I did not know. Some had traveled quite a distance and some were neighbors. I was surprised by the small turnout, but then, it's a small church and a small town.

As we all slowly filed into the sanctuary filling up our allotted number of pews directly in front of the pulpit, I knew the congregation was looking us over, attempting to assess how we were all holding up. As usual, I was doing the poorest job.

Mother's grandchildren were her pallbearers. Michael, the oldest, was in charge of the urn, and Aaron, the youngest, led the processional carrying a large, gold cross. The pastor's words were genuine and kind. He spoke about all of us, her church family and how happy she was now that she was with her heavenly family. He sounded so sure of himself, but I didn't feel so sure of such things. I wanted to believe in heaven and a reunion with my mother someday but found myself questioning the very idea of God and heaven. I don't think anyone else in my family did. They were all more faithful believers than me. I wondered if my mother had doubts too, especially at the end. I was glad the pastor acknowledged living without her would be hard. I was impressed with his compassion, especially since he didn't know Mother very well, being new to the church and also since I remembered those obscenities she had tossed his way during their recent visit. He seemed to sense I was having a lot of difficulty holding it together as he repeatedly made direct eye contact with me when he was giving his sermon, or maybe he knew in those moments I was the weakest believer.

Later at the cemetery, Peter and Aaron placed the urn into the vault in the ground. It was comforting to have them involved. What a remarkable memory for them, placing Grandma's ashes in their final resting place. Lindsay and Josh stood nearby. Dad held up well, but his sadness was a tangible thing. Again, he patted my arm as we stood there looking at Mother's grave. I tried to imagine what it must feel like saying goodbye to someone you shared your life with for almost 60 years.

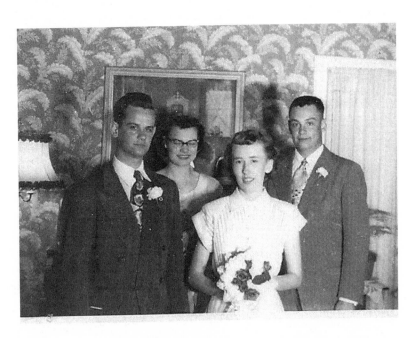

My parents on their wedding day, June 8, 1950. I always thought it was so sweet they were married on my mother's birthday.

The March wind felt even colder at the cemetery. Unsure of how long they should stay, people slowly started leaving, carefully avoiding the muddiest spots and patches of snow and ice that remained.

After the church luncheon, we spent the rest of the afternoon back at Dad's socializing with people who stopped by, one group arranging itself around the dining room table and another group of people sitting uncomfortably close to one another in the living room. Susan, Kay and I dutifully set out plates full of sandwiches, bars and cookies that no one really seemed interested in eating. No one talked much about Mother, which I found odd, even irritating. Instead there was meaningless conversation about unimportant things like the weather, basketball games and food.

Susan, Kay and I walked around the house reminiscing and peeking into rooms, almost whispering to each other as if we might come upon Mother somewhere.

The afternoon ended with tired, awkward goodbyes on the front porch. People didn't really know when to leave or what to say when they did. Death makes things so awkward.

Later as we made the three-hour drive back home to Wisconsin, I thought about a lot of things, but said little. I had no idea how I was supposed to carry on without a mother. One thing I knew for sure was I had crossed the bridge for good now; there was no going back to my old life, the one in which I had a mother. Luckily, I brought bits and pieces of her with me to keep forever as treasures of my heart. I was a different person, a motherless daughter and forever changed, but at the same time, still very much my mother's daughter.

-32-

Chemo

July 13 – day one

My alarm blares at 4:20 a.m.

It feels like deja vu as I shower and put on my brown terrycloth sweatpants and sweatshirt, the same outfit I wore to my bilateral mastectomy six weeks ago. I guess it's now my surgery outfit. Today I am having the freaking port put in. Oh, and I'm also beginning chemo. Shit. How did this become my life?

David and I arrive at the hospital feeling like we really have this surgery routine down. Once I am settled into my pre-op room and things are given the go-ahead, I relax a bit, but just a bit. This procedure must be considered pretty minor as no chaplain makes an appearance this time. All the other rig-a-ma-role is pretty much the same. When someone deems it's time, once again I am wheeled away and headed for the OR.

Waking up this time from anesthesia is a snap, thank God; it's nothing like the last time. Upon awakening I remember nothing but notice I have a blanket over my face and for a brief instant wonder if I've died. Luckily, I can still breathe. I listen to the activity and am soon directed to move myself to the gurney, and we then head back to my room for a brief recovery period. Next, we receive some debriefing and directions from our nurse, and then I am sent on my way up to the infamous fifth floor, the oncology floor. I am required to ride in a strange wheelchair-like contraption, pushed by a young volunteer who seems unsure about how to get up to the fifth floor. I decide I will make no effort to help direct her. I'm certainly in no hurry to get up there. Who cares if we get lost for a bit?

Eventually, of course, we make our way to the proper floor and David is already there waiting. We are greeted warmly by a blond-haired nurse with a pleasant personality. I'm glad it's not the chemo class nurse from hell.

We get to choose which chemo room we want because things are pretty slow so far this morning. We decide on the quieter room with only one other chemo recipient in it at the moment. The other room seems way too noisy with too many people, too much talking and too many televisions blaring. I choose a brown, leather recliner that feels surprisingly pretty comfortable. I suppose it's actually vinyl, not leather. I sit down feeling calmer than I thought I would be. The room is fairly small with a wood floor, about five other chemo recliners, a small television and too many outdated magazines stacked on a table. There are two small windows on one wall, but they are too high up and the blinds are pulled shut, so there's no view. There are large glass windows so nurses can keep an eye on us sitting in here as they pass by in the hallway, not unlike peering at animals behind the glass at a zoo. Memories of sitting beside Mother when she had chemo flood back to me, and I am overwhelmed with the concept I am in need of such a thing merely two years later. It seems incredibly absurd, ridiculous and just plain unbelievable I am now sitting in a chemo chair. How the hell did this happen?

David sits next to me on an uncomfortable-looking, basic folding chair with no arm rests. I guess his comfort isn't as much of a concern to the staff. He looks uneasy and I wonder what he's thinking. We wait for the next nurse to gather my chemo cocktail supplies and just keep looking at each other with worried eyes. This nurse is very kind too. Her name is Karla. She explains everything she is doing slowly and compassionately.

"Is this your first time?" she asks.

"Yes," I answer.

"Are you nervous?"

"I just want to get it over with," I answer.

First she administers an anti-nausea solution. About thirty minutes later she returns with two vials of bright red fluid which she slowly injects into the IV unit. The bright red fluid is the Red Devil itself, Adriamycin. I want to vomit.

"Now I'm really nervous," I tell her.

Watching the red poison entering my body is horrifying, but what choice do I have? I feel powerless. I also receive Cytoxin. This one is clear and not quite as intimidating in appearance anyway.

Finally, after about two hours we are finished, I am unhooked and we head for the door after reviewing our going home instructions with Nurse Karla. I need to take more medication to prevent nausea. I must stay on top of things to avoid that. Believe me, I plan to. Before stepping into the elevator, I stop at the restroom. My urine is a startling red color, just as I had been warned it would be. This makes me feel vampire-like.

The rest of the day passes and I begin to relax somewhat, thankful the first round is over. I wait for side effects to kick in, but I don't feel too badly or much different. What I do feel is exhausted, mentally as much as physically.

July 15

I can't sleep at night due to the steroids and anti-nausea pills. I wake up at 2:30 a.m. and move to the blue, leather sofa in the family room, but I can't sleep there either, or even get comfortable. Water tastes incredibly metallic and nasty, and I struggle to swallow it. I force myself to do it because I know I must. Water is supposed to flush these toxins out of my body, but what if I flush them out too quickly before they get their cancer cell killing job finished? Drinking water makes me feel like gagging but being constipated is worse, so I drink it anyway. Drinking milk is out of the question.

July 17

It's day five into chemo. The road ahead feels endless. I'm not even sure how many days there are in sixteen weeks. I avoid doing the math to figure it out. Regardless, it's too many days. I don't know if I can get through today much less sixteen weeks. I hate this shit.

David and I drive to Woodbury one more time so I can try on the two wigs we ordered in different colors and then pick the best one.

It's a good thing we started this process weeks ago as I can hardly function mentally. Only one color even remotely works, so this decision is an easy one. I cannot wait to get out of the store, but I do feel relieved to have my two wigs purchased. I also decided to buy a few scarves, caps and a halo, which is a band you can wear that has fake hair all around it, creating a halo effect. What a stupid name for it though.

July 18

How do I feel now as a person on chemo? Honestly, I feel as if I am consumed by it. It seems my life can now be divided into pre-chemo days, chemo days and one day soon hopefully post-chemo days. I think about chemo and cancer a lot. I feel engulfed by it. Sometimes it's hard to think about other things and realize other people have thoughts about things not related to cancer at all. It's as if I am living in a different world where I do not belong. I quite literally live in Cancer Land now and I hate it here. The other day I heard someone on TV say she was grateful for the "opportunity" cancer gave her to grow. What the fuck?

Luckily, I am not nauseous at all and I am so grateful for this. I feel like there is a veil over me, or like I am a wild animal trapped in a net and I can't escape no matter how much I struggle. I am captured. Maybe this is how people who do drugs feel, kind of spacy and mentally shaky. I can feel dramatic changes taking place in my body, almost as if I can actually detect my cells fighting amongst themselves to determine which ones will live and which ones will die. It's very weird. Surprisingly, I am hungry much of the time. If I don't eat every two hours or so, I start to feel like I'm starving. I must eat something, no ifs, ands or buts about it. At the same time, it's scary to eat, too, because I never know for sure how something will taste or if it will upset my stomach. Eating is a balancing act now, something requiring timing, precision, the right quantities and luck. Oh, and let's not forget shopping, preparing and cleaning up, which thankfully my family is mostly taking care of.

All in all, I feel okay, just not like myself. I don't remember what I used to feel like. That person seems lost forever, as if she fell through a trap door. I am starting to wonder if she will ever be found or seen again.

July 19

Today it appears I am in phase two of the chemo cycle. Now I have diarrhea which scares me. I am afraid to eat.

July 20

One week on chemo and I'm still here. I have to get some blood drawn today so my counts can be checked. A nurse calls this afternoon to inform me that yes, they are low.

"Be sure to wash your hands extra often and avoid sick people," she advises.

It's scary to realize my body is in such a vulnerable state, especially since one week ago my counts were all normal. Fucking with the body's natural immune system seems wrong. I hope the medical people know what the hell they're doing.

July 22

I finally feel pretty good again. I even have normal bowels. I used to think Mother was nuts to be so darn concerned about her bowel movements. Now I totally get it.

July 27 – round two

Wouldn't you know it, just when I am starting to feel better it's time to go back for round two of chemo. First we must meet with Dr. Nambudiri.

"How have things been going for you?" his nurse asks.

"Oh, pretty well," I say.

I try not to complain about my side effects too much, though why this is I do not know. There is so much pretending that goes on in Cancer Land. Why is this? Who are we protecting?

The appointment with Dr. Nambudiri goes well. We don't arrive with so many questions anymore which I guess means we are figuring this shit out.

"Your blood counts have recovered nicely," he says.

This is a relief.

"During the nadir, the three day period of each chemo cycle when your white counts are low, you must be very careful about being around sick people and call us immediately if you have any fever or symptoms of infection," he says.

It's not so much what he says but how he says it that frightens me. His words make me feel even more vulnerable and emphasize how little control I have over my own body. I am in a fragile state, and I don't like it.

We head for our preferred chemo room, the quiet one, but today it isn't quiet. There is only one recliner left, so I head over to take my seat before someone else grabs it. Who knew a chemo room could be a place where you have to quickly claim your spot? I envision fights breaking out over recliners. That could get interesting.

Today my chemo nurse irritates me. She's obviously a talker. I am not, especially when sitting in a God damn chemo chair. I should tell her to be quiet, but I don't want to be rude.

"I do so admire you patients for returning and choosing more treatment. It's a choice you know. You don't have to be here," she says.

What the fuck?

Hearing this pisses me off more. I know she means well, so again, I keep quiet. She does bring me a nice warm blanket which feels heavenly, so maybe she's not so bad after all.

"This drug is super toxic," she says. "This is why we wear these special robes and protect ourselves in case some should drip on us. If it gets on your skin or out of your bloodstream, it can eat away at skin, tissue and organs."

Great, I think to myself; that's a nice visual you're giving me. It's terrifying to think of this bright red fluid flowing through my veins intermingling with my blood and unsuspecting healthy cells, an ambush of sorts. It makes sense to require poison to kill those bastardly cancer cells. It doesn't make quite as much sense to kill healthy cells at the same time.

When my two hours are up, I can't wait to get out of my chair, find the emergency door, which they allow chemo patients to use to exit, and head for home. Makes sense to let us use the emergency door because getting out of here does feel like a God damn emergency. I can't get out the door fast enough. I can't get home fast enough either.

-33-

Fall Out

July 28 – two weeks & one day in

My hair is starting to fall out. While showering this morning it seemed I was losing more, but maybe I was just imagining it. Maybe I won't be shampooing my hair too many more times in the near future. There's a timetable here too, another thing about cancer and chemo that is so damn predictable. I try to imagine what I will look like bald, with no hair at all. I can't. Picturing such a thing seems unimaginable.

July 29

The hairs on my brush and the ones on the back of my shirt confirm to me that yes, my hair is falling out. I carefully pick them off my shirt and wonder how fast it will happen. Even though this is totally expected, I'm not ready. Who would be?

I walk into the family room where David is watching TV and sit down on the blue, leather sofa.

"Well, you better take one last look at me with hair because it's starting," I announce.

What a dumb thing to say.

"I'm sorry," David says.

The look in his eyes says a whole lot more. He looks at me with such genuine love, concern, empathy and compassion. I notice what his face also shows is a look of utter helplessness, for there is nothing he can do this time. This is a new look, a more intense look, one that makes me suddenly realize I must try not to be such a baby about losing my hair, not only for my sake, but for his as well. Not until this moment did I realize how worried he has been about this hair loss thing too.

July 30

My hair is coming out at a pretty good clip now. Wow, isn't that a stupid pun? I guess I must be pretty vain about my hair. So many women say when they begin losing their hair, they make a beeline to their hairdresser and get it shaved off right away. I've even heard about some throwing a hair-shaving party. That is so not for me. Why would I want to turn this nightmare into some weird kind of party? And why would I want to hurry the process along? It makes me feel like I'm doing the hair loss thing all wrong. It makes me feel like I'm doing cancer wrong.

Maybe I'm an oddball, but I want the process to linger. I am in no hurry. I carefully, and yes, sometimes tearfully, pull out the loose hairs dangling around my shoulders as they drop out. I meticulously remove strands clinging to my clothes as if saying goodbye to old friends. If someone was watching me, they'd probably think, what a silly woman, but I don't care. This is how I feel more in control. Sometimes my head feels itchy, and I run outside and start feverishly brushing. I watch the hairs float away in the breeze.

It doesn't really matter how you do this hair loss thing. Shave it off, or let it happen slowly; when all is said and done, you end up bald.

July 31

My new reaction after round two of chemo is flushing. When I saw myself in the mirror yesterday and again when I looked today, my face, neck, chest and back are red and a pretty bright red at that. I look like I have a bad sunburn, and it's a startling thing to see. Flushing is caused by dilating capillaries, just another thing screwed up by chemotherapy. My chest also feels super tight, so I find myself hoping and praying my expanders are okay. It feels as if I am about to explode. On the up side, the dang metallic taste seems to be somewhat better. Now if only I could sleep at night. I have forgotten what a good night's sleep feels like too. It's horribly ironic to feel so incredibly tired but at the same time be unable to sleep through the night. A person's body on chemo is totally fucked up. Totally.

-34-

Scourge

Cancer is a scourge. I read that in a magazine today and just reading it made me feel badly. I don't like being part of a scourge. Who would? Even the word sounds thorny and evil. But cancer is evil. It's like a serpent waiting to strike and swallow you whole. Or maybe it's more like a science-fiction-type virus that methodically takes over your body in unsuspecting tiny increments until it mutates into an unstoppable force, attempting to consume its victim's body bit by bit. In the beginning, you don't even know you're host to such a thing. The cancer is never satisfied but always hungry for more. It seems cunning and overpowering, taking pieces of you away and tricking you into believing you have rid yourself of it, when in reality, you are just waiting for the other shoe to drop. You think you are recovering from your latest assignment of cancer duties—the diagnosis, the biopsy, the surgery, the chemo, but really you are only in a waiting game. It's like some kind of "chess match" between you and cancer. You're never quite sure you have made the right moves or if you ever will. The stakes of this match are high; it's not win or lose but live or die.

How do I feel now as a person on chemo? A good way to describe it is that I feel like Dr. Jekyll and Mr. Hyde, as if I have a split personality. My two-week chemo cycle is split right down the middle. For the first week, especially the first five days, I am basically miserable with little sleep, a metallic taste in my mouth, intense flushing and zero energy. I'm supposed to be grateful for not feeling nauseous and I am, but still, even without the nausea chemo completely sucks. My mind and thoughts are cloudy and fuzzy. I find myself falling asleep while sitting in a chair watching TV. I can sleep, wake up, go directly to bed and fall asleep again. There's no such thing as too much sleep, but yet I rarely sleep through the night, so go figure. I get hungry, and often, but no food tastes particularly good, so eating is not very pleasant, sad but true. Even less enjoyable is drinking the necessary fluids. Sometimes drinking water makes me gag, but I know I must drink it anyway. Around day four, I am incredibly moody, which really means crabby. I also cry at the drop of a hat. Basically, I'm a mess. A bitchy mess at that.

By about day six, I am starting to feel considerably better and more like my old self. Each night I sleep a bit better as well. I am starting to really appreciate the better days of the second week in the cycle. Once in a while I even forget I am on chemo, until I look in the mirror. The image I see looking back is an instant reminder. Still, I love those moments when I do forget. I'll try to avoid mirrors.

It's super hard to return to the next scheduled chemo session when you are starting to feel better. Just when your body is adapting, successfully rebuilding and bouncing back, you throw it back into the wringer for more punishment. The words of that chemo nurse echo in my mind, the ones about me making the choice to come back each time for more. Yeah, like I have a choice. Choosing chemo does not make me a person to admire, nor does it mean I am strong. In fact, it would take a stronger-willed person to rebel and choose a less proven treatment path.

What I might be is resilient, or rather, my body is anyway. After experiencing firsthand how my body struggles and works so hard to resurge itself time and time again, I am filled with a deep appreciation for its ability to regenerate and renew. It truly is miraculous. Yes, resilient, that's what I am. I'll go with that.

-35-

A Wedding

August 14 – one month in

Today is my niece's wedding day. I have been looking forward to this day but have also been feeling apprehensive about it. A wedding is an event to be anticipated, celebrated and enjoyed. It's normally a joyous occasion, but when you have cancer, even weddings can feel awkward and make you feel anxious for all kinds of reasons.

This is the second wedding in my family cancer has fucked around with.

Luckily, I had a decent night's sleep last night so at least I start the day feeling relatively good. Peter and Aaron will drive separately to Madelia in case I don't feel up to staying for the entire day and want to come home early. When undergoing chemo, you must be prepared for worst-case scenarios. You must always have a backup plan.

Getting myself physically ready takes considerable effort and more than a bit of time. I carefully apply my makeup, attempting to look presentable and at least somewhat like my former self. I'm grateful I still have a few eyelashes so I can put my mascara wand to work. What I really need is a fairy godmother's magic wand to transform me. Wouldn't that be nice? My outfit is satisfactory at best. The final step is plopping on my wig and combing my fake bob's stray hairs into place. Upon completion of my makeover, I gaze into the mirror feeling more like a secret agent attending a wedding in disguise than

163

an aunt of the bride. I decide I look alright, just not entirely like myself. Actually, not at all like myself. I hope the day will not be too hot, but of course the forecast calls for high heat and humidity. Shit.

The wedding takes place in an old-fashioned country church that Kay and Tim belong to located near their hog farm. Of course, it has no air-conditioning. The church is surrounded by cornfields, with a gravel road leading up to it, as if frozen in an earlier time period. Its walls hold secrets of countless other weddings, funerals, confirmations and baptisms. It looks beautiful with its white, wooden, hand-carved altar, intricate paintings of Jesus hanging on the walls and creaking stairways full of whispers from the past.

We sit down on the padded pews unsuccessfully trying to stay cool and wait for the bride to walk down the aisle. I'm even more eager to see Lindsay; she's a bridesmaid. The wedding begins right on time, the ceremony led by a young, blond minister who for no real reason seems out of place in such an old, rural church setting.

Lindsay looks beautiful and elegant in her purple, strapless dress and silver shoes. She walks gracefully and slowly down the aisle accompanied by her assigned groomsman appearing totally at ease. Rachel, the bride, looks lovely as well as she makes her way down the aisle, and I remember the two giggling, skinny girls who made up silly games and spent hours searching for and naming dust bunnies. Today they are confident young women. David and I sit side by side listening to words about commitment and marriage through sickness and health, something the two standing at the altar probably know little about. David and I know a thing or two about these things. We have endured, even through cancer. In this, at least, I am lucky.

After the ceremony, I decide I do feel up to going to the reception. I feel a need to show up. Cancer will not decide what I do or do not do, not today.

It's an odd feeling to know many people attending today's wedding don't know me and have no idea I have breast cancer. When I greet them and shake their hands, they have no idea the woman under the wig has cancer and actually looks much different. I am an imposter. Others do know and more than likely are looking me over for signs of something amiss. Or perhaps I only image they do. Regardless, it doesn't matter. I am a sister to the mother of the bride. I showed up. I functioned. I contributed. I made a difference. I smiled. It was a hard day, but it was also a good day. But damn, I'm tired.

-36-

Treading Water, Anger & Cancer Bullshit

Step by step we are making our way through this tidal wave that is chemo. Some days the waves feel unmanageably powerful, and I feel I am being pulled under and will surely sink. I keep trying to come up for air but can't quite make it. Just when the wave begins to recede, it's time to return for another round of poisoning, and today it's time for round four. I must try to stay afloat. I am treading water and I hate it. I wonder if other patients have such disdain for chemo. I doubt it. No one could hate it this much.

The fourth treatment wipes me out. I am exhausted. And now it's time to start worrying about the next round when I change poisons. Just when you start to figure stuff out, they change things up on you.

Today I am out of breath and my flushing has returned making me look as if I've spent too much time at the beach. My chest is tight. Everything tastes bad, even chocolate. I make chocolate chip cookies and even they taste weird, and I only eat one. You'd think I'd be losing weight, but I'm not. I am lethargic, bloated, ugly and cranky. I wonder if everyone wants to stay away from me. I'd sure like to if I could. I'm an emotional mess.

I've decided a person with cancer can experience a wide range of emotions on a daily basis. No, wait, it's more like on an hourly basis or even a minute-to-minute basis. Emotional turbulence, that's what it is. A few emotions that arise without warning at times are fear, uncertainty, vulnerability, anxiousness, disgust, despair, loneliness and anger. Perhaps the two most powerful of these are fear and anger. I don't feel fear as much these days, so maybe this indicates anger is stronger because I still get plenty angry fairly often. I've also decided this is not necessarily a bad thing.

When I first received the phone call from the asshole doctor who gave me my diagnosis, I was angry. He delivered the news matter-of-factly. He did not convey a feeling of empathy or urgency, and that made me angry. I was angry cancer chose me. I was angry the disease of breast cancer still existed. I was angry for not taking better care of myself. I was angry I had not had genetic testing yet. I was angry for getting cancer decades younger than Mother. I was angry with her for not being here when I needed her most. I was angry for being the one to put David and my kids in this predicament, a situation they did not deserve to be in. I was angry at cancer for interrupting the smoothness of my life, for changing its course, for just butting in where it did not belong. Yeah, I was darn angry. So what?

Anger, just like any emotion, isn't good or bad. It's just another one you sometimes need to feel. It's like a pot of boiling water on a stove. The water starts off at a slow simmer, with gentle bubbles creating a little bit of heat and steam. It becomes hotter, more intense and then dangerous. If the water continues to boil, eventually it dissipates and you end up with nothing but a burnt, ill-smelling pot.

Anger can simmer, too, until it eventually "boils" over, leaving you feeling empty and burned out. If you allow yourself to feel your anger and use its power for something constructive, then it can be useful. It can make you want to get off your ass and get things done.

Besides, isn't any emotion valid if you are feeling it? Guess not. Some emotions are not allowed in Cancer Land, and anger seems to be one of them. This is total bullshit to me. Why do we have emotions such as anger if we are not "allowed" to tap into them. In the long run, feeling your anger might actually be essential to your well-being. A person can't keep turning herself inside out trying to stomp out genuine feelings, not if she wants to avoid an "explosion" down the road anyway. Plus, it's too exhausting. If anyone deserves to feel angry from time to time, it's someone with cancer, and probably her caregiver too.

I'm noticing my cancer pet peeves are beginning to pile up. Certain aspects of all this cancer mumbo-jumbo are just plain annoying. There is so much bullshit out there in Cancer Land, especially in Breast Cancer Land; it's actually quite remarkable. There could be a book written just about breast cancer bullshit. My biggest pet peeve by far is hearing some people say how cancer has changed their life for the better, and they are actually grateful for this "gift." Are you kidding me? Some gift. I will not give cancer credit for making me into a better person either. I'm not. In fact, I might have gone the other direction. I fear I very well might be far less patient, more cynical and less willing to conform, especially to proper cancer etiquette. I'm not exactly sure what this is, but there seem to be many out there professing to know the right way to "do" cancer. It's like there's some kind of cancer handbook, and if you don't follow it just right, people think you're uncooperative, negative or ungrateful.

Of course, I understand what some might mean when they say some of this stuff. At least I think I do. They probably mean they appreciate life more after a diagnosis, look at things differently and generally have a fresh perspective on things. Cancer can be a wake-up call. But guess what? I didn't need cancer to make me appreciate my life and my family. I was doing just fine in those departments before cancer came along. I appreciated both before and I appreciate them now. I did not need enlightenment, thank you very much. Have I learned some things? Of course I have, but I would have learned things had I not had cancer too. Before cancer I tried to learn from what was going on around me. After cancer, I try to learn from whatever is going on around me. I tried to be a better person every day before cancer. And I still shoot for that now. So why should cancer get any credit for any of it?

Another pet peeve I have is regarding all that brave and strong cancer language bullshit. I am not strong. I am not brave. In fact, I really don't want anything to do with that whole cancer warrior notion. I am not and never will be a cancer-ass-kicking-warrior type of gal. That's just not the way I roll. And yes, sometimes I feel like a cancer failure because of this. I do not feel, look or act like the tough, cancer-fighting shero all decked out in pink who vows to kick cancer to the curb. I guess someone like that is supposed to be the shining example of how to do this crap. I can't be that person. I don't want to be that person.

And as for all the other war metaphors, I have no time for those either. No time whatsoever. It is so much more complicated than just fighting hard. What about the people with cancer, like my mother, who gave their all but died anyway? Did they not "fight the battle" hard enough? Was it their fault they died? This is the message in such talk, even if unintended isn't it?

And then there is the constant pressure to above all else, just stay positive. As if the answer to everything, including cancer, is to keep smiling. What a crock that is. My mother was a very positive person, and that did not save her. Being positive is fine and dandy when you feel up to it, but when you don't, feeling that pressure to hide your true feelings can be a very heavy burden to carry around on this already stressful and difficult enough cancer gig, which, by the way, is not a journey. I will not be calling it that. A journey is something you plan for, pack for and enjoy. And you get to pick your destination. Calling cancer a journey trivializes a disease experience, making it sound more like a Hallmark made-for-TV movie with a predictable beginning, middle and end. Cancer is not predictable. At all. Cancer sucks. Pure and simple. And I do not intend to smile my way through it. Everything in life is not meant to be turned into something positive, and it seems to me cancer might be one of these things. Everything does not happen for a reason either, nor are you necessarily only given what you can handle. More bullshit. Sometimes shitty stuff just happens, and you try to muddle your way through as best you can. Some days I want to shout from my rooftop or grab a microphone and yell to the world, cancer sucks! Because it does.

And one more thing, I'm waiting for my epiphany moment, that moment when things (what things I do not know) become clear to me. Why must there be great life lessons learned from cancer anyway? Isn't this just one more attempt to frame it as a gift?

I would argue that cancer is a great hands-on teacher of mostly shitty stuff. Sure, perhaps you pick up a few nuggets of wisdom along the way, but I'd rather by-pass the rendezvous with cancer and be less enlightened. Who needs the kind of wisdom you garner from cancer? Who needs this kind of "gift"?

I am becoming a rebellious sort of cancer patient. Who knew?

-37-

Bald *Is* *Not* *All* that *Beautiful*

Miraculously, we somehow make it through October, and I finally finish up chemo. You might think I'd be dancing in the streets about now, but I'm not—not yet anyway. Don't get me wrong, I'm totally thrilled to be finished with the nightmare that is chemo. I hated everything about it, except of course, the fact it was killing off remaining stubborn cancer cells just trying to find a secret, safe place in my body to hunker down, hide out and wait for the opportunity to start doing their damage all over again.

When I finished chemo the other day, the nurses gave me a certificate which was meant to be a validation of some sort that I had survived, come out on the other side or whatever. When they handed it to me, all I wanted to do was rush home and tear it to shreds. Of course, instead I just smiled and thanked them because I knew their intentions were completely admirable and I was grateful—very grateful. Still, I just couldn't grasp the idea of that dang certificate. I also got a bottle of some kind of sparkling apple juice. Now *that* I appreciated.

Now that chemo's over, I finally gave in and shaved off the rest of my hair the other night, or I should say, David shaved it off for me. Even though I was definitely ready and didn't even have much hair remaining to shave off, it was still a difficult and emotional thing for both of us to experience. My tears started flowing pretty freely. David silently buzzed while I wondered what he was thinking. This sure as heck isn't what he signed up for either.

Today someone said to me, it's only hair. It'll grow back in no time. I wanted to smack that person. It's not just hair and losing it is a big deal and no, it doesn't grow back in no time. I don't trust anyone who says this kind of stuff, though of course they mean well and I should probably cut them some slack, but not now. Maybe later.

I am glad I waited to go bald until the end of chemo, rather than shaving off my hair early on. For me, that was the right time. Many people don't realize your entire body often can and does go "bald" with many chemo regimens. It's really weird to not have hair under your arms, on your legs or in your private area. Even the little nose hairs disappear, which was quite shocking for me to realize one day when I couldn't figure out why my nose kept running. That was one of those "duh" moments.

When I think of all the physical changes my body has gone through over the past few months, it's pretty staggering. It certainly gives a whole new meaning to the saying, beauty is in the eye of the beholder. I used to think my hair was one of my best features. When I was in high school and college, most girls had long, straight hair and mine was as well. My friends frequently mentioned they liked my hair, even though I'm pretty sure mine looked about the same as theirs. In more recent years, my hair started thinning a bit and turning gray. I started coloring it and it looked alright, but it was no longer my best feature. Today when I look at recent pictures of myself, I marvel at how much hair I had, and I'm pretty darn envious of how I looked just a few months ago. I miss the old me in more ways than one. I want her back.

After my hair, I have always considered my eyes to be my next best feature, or at least I worked hard at trying to make them that. I started wearing mascara in seventh or eighth grade, which adds up to lots of tubes of black mascara over the years. These days I squint when looking in the mirror trying to even see my sparse eyelashes. It seems pointless attempting to curl them and to apply mascara, which only seems to clump onto two lashes per eye. Not a good look.

Then there is the rest of my body between my neck and ankles. Needless to say, after a bilateral mastectomy with ongoing reconstruction, I look nothing like I once did in this region either.

This gets me down to my feet. Along with my hands, they are pretty much the only body parts that haven't changed much over the past months. Oh wait, my feet are still numb from the neuropathy, but hopefully this will improve. At least my fingernails and toenails never fell off from chemo. Some chemo patients aren't so lucky.

I try not to judge people anymore by their appearances. Judging others based on their looks goes on a lot in our society. Of course, I always tried not to do this before cancer, but now I am super serious about trying to never do it again. Beautiful qualities within people are indeed what matter most. We need to look beneath that outer layer. This is a simple truth most of us believe but also one we mostly give lip service to.

Now that I'm bald, I'm finding it even less fun to look in the mirror. Sometimes I think this makes me shallow, but really it's because looking at my reflection now is so startling. My "best" features are no more. I hardly recognize the person staring back at me, and sometimes I ask right out loud, *who is that?*

And just for the record, bald is not all that beautiful, at least not on this body.

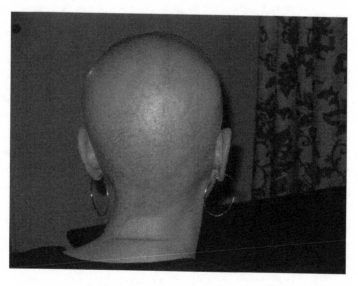

I did not embrace my baldness. I hated it & sometimes felt I was doing cancer all wrong because of this. Now I know better.

-38-

The Swap

Today is December 2 and it's time for the swap. It's time to undergo another surgery to replace these uncomfortable expanders with new, unfamiliar silicone implants. I'm swapping one set of fakes for another set of fakes. Swap day takes me back to last spring shortly after my diagnosis. Sitting in a plastic surgeon's office that day felt surreal. I never imagined myself needing a plastic surgeon. Not me. I would grow older and wiser welcoming (okay, trying to welcome) wrinkles, sagging jowls and everything else gravity eventually takes down with it. But there David and I sat, once again making decisions about things we never planned to deal with. We passed around sample silicone gel implants as if replacing my real breasts with them was no big deal

A month or so ago when my plastic surgeon and I were discussing a date for this latest procedure, he threw out a few other dates including December 2. The minute I heard he was available on December 2, that's the date I wanted. By choosing this date, *exactly* six months out from my bilateral date, I was making a statement. I'm not exactly sure what sort of statement but a statement nonetheless.

When I reflect upon the last six months, I am amazed at what my body has endured. Even more amazing, perhaps, is how both David and I have adjusted to the whole mastectomy thing. I guess when you are facing life and death, breasts suddenly fall way below life on the scale of importance.

This is not to say any of this has been easy. It hasn't. It's been hell at times. And today I am having more than a few doubts, not about the mastectomy, but about the implants. Maybe I should be satisfied to not bother with implants at all. Maybe I should have researched more about DIEP flap, TRAM flap and other various flap procedures. Maybe I should be putting in smaller implants. Maybe I should be putting in larger ones. Why are silicone implants deemed safe now? Weren't they banned a few years back? And what will I do about nipples and tattoos? Still so many questions and worries, when will it all end? I'm so tired of it all. And I have a case of cold feet. Any surgery is scary. I need to just get on with it and get this part over with too. It's one more step I need to take.

Before heading into the OR, I meet with my plastic surgeon to address a few concerns. It's never too late for that—or too late to opt out, but I don't. While speaking with him one more time about the proper implant size for me, he makes a few more marks on my chest with his black marker. My chest has become a drawing board.

"Our team will be sitting you up for a bit when you're on the operating table to help us better determine what size implant will work best for you," he says.

What am I supposed to say to that?

Of course, he and I have discussed size before, but this will be the final analysis. It freaks me out a little knowing I will be literally sized up while out cold, but what the hell, it's one more indignation to withstand. At least I won't have to listen to the conversation. Thank God.

After about a two-hour procedure which also included the removal of my chemo port by my other surgeon (hurray!), I spend another hour or so in recovery and another thirty minutes back in the post-op room. By 1 p.m. David and I are sent on our way with ice packs, discharge directions and phone numbers. It seems pretty amazing to have surgery in the morning and head home the same afternoon. Once home I head straight for the blue, leather sofa. Again.

I have little pain this time. Compared to my bilateral mastectomy this feels like a piece of cake. Okay, not quite, but sort of. I will still need to sleep on my back for the time being, but I've become pretty used to this position since tissue expanders. I wonder if I'll ever be able to sleep on my stomach again. I miss that so much. It was always my best sleeping position, just another thing lost.

Sleeping on your back is supposedly good for wrinkle prevention. You don't wake up with dents on your face from your pillow. When I visited my Grandma Clara every summer when growing up, she often took a nap in the afternoon, and when she got up, her face looked squished and wrinkled in places. I'd stare at and study her face, unable to comprehend the reason for such a thing. Now I get it. I read an article about Michelle Pfeiffer once in a magazine in which she stated one of her beauty secrets was sleeping on her back for this exact reason, to prevent wrinkles. It seems to work for her, so maybe it will for me too.

I am relieved to be done with yet another step in this cancer shitstorm. I still have more steps ahead. I still have more surgery. I still have more worries, some of which I don't even know about yet. I cannot worry about things that are ahead. I cannot worry about potential worries. Or can I? Cancer is really all about worry. Worry, worry, worry. Enough. There is only so much worrying a person's mind can handle at a time. All I can do is keep moving forward. And this is enough.

-39-

Next Level & a Vacation from Myself

A Christmas tree in a hospital lobby looks so out of place. You can decorate it and make it look quite lovely, but it's still a Christmas tree in a hospital lobby for crying out loud. It just doesn't fit in.

As I make my way past the Christmas tree, into the elevator and on up to the now too familiar fifth floor, the cancer floor, I am struck by how calm I am. I've arrived for my first oncology checkup. My perception about the hospital atmosphere has evolved in the months since my diagnosis, yet it has not. I have adjusted and yet I have not. I feel comfortable on the fifth floor, yet I do not. I feel like that towering Christmas tree in the lobby. Just like the tree, I'm trying hard to fit in here, but I don't and I never will.

In the past, standing in line waiting for my turn to check in made me feel as if I were being scrutinized by the other patients. I felt like everyone could tell I had cancer. I felt like I stuck out. Now I realize how ridiculous that feeling was. First of all, no one else was ever focused on me; they all had problems of their own. Secondly, even if everyone knew I had cancer, in that particular waiting room, such a fact did not make me stand out anyway, sad but true.

I check in with the familiar face at the appointment registration desk. The receptionist asks me the same questions she always asks, and I robotically answer them like I always do. I still get that same feeling I had in the ER on the day of the mass sighting, like I'm being sized up and evaluated by the person behind the counter too. And

175

then I go sit down to wait, and there's more sizing up being done by everyone else who's sitting on waiting room chairs. But then there's not much else to do in waiting rooms, especially in cancer waiting rooms.

Like everyone else, I sit and observe the patients coming and going too. I wonder at what point each of them is in their diagnosis or treatment. I observe some obviously new patients busily filling out forms with worried expressions on their faces, uncertain of their futures. Others sit patiently with their scarves, wigs or hats camouflaging their bare heads while waiting for their next chemo infusion. One or two sit surrounded by uncomfortable-looking family members reminding me of the many appointments I accompanied Mother on. One paces around the room, unable to wait quietly in his seat, much like a fidgety student in one of my classrooms.

Familiar-looking nurses appear every few minutes to collect the next patients on their lists. One or two of them acknowledge me with a smile or nod, recognizing my face as someone who has gone through the "cancer program" and graduated to the next level. Clearly, they are busily occupied with their newest "class."

When it's my turn and my name is called, the old familiar feeling of disbelief kicks in. Even after all these months I can't believe I need an oncologist and maybe always will. I can't believe I was diagnosed with breast cancer. I can't believe I tested positive for the darn gene mutation, endured a bilateral mastectomy, completed a huge chunk of reconstruction and recently finished chemotherapy. Is this really my life?

While these unpleasant memories are permanently etched into my memory, I still can't believe such memories belong to me. In some ways I still feel as disconnected to cancer as I did on the day of my diagnosis. It still feels unreal. I wonder if this will ever change.

"I still can't believe I need an oncologist," I mention.

"Well, you do," David says.

At times it continues to feel as if I'm observing someone else's life. Are such thoughts normal? Am I still too close to it all with not enough time elapsed yet? Is it some kind of strange mind game? Am I not progressing properly? Am I a cancer failure? Does everyone in this "cancer program" feel like this? I have no answers to much of anything these days. I'm still stuck in the maze that is cancer. Will I ever find my way out?

David and I make it through the appointment successfully, limiting our list of questions to only a page so as not to overwhelm any of us. I have advanced to the next level and don't need to come back for three whole months. It's too bad you can't ever graduate for good from the cancer program. Once you're in this blankety-blank program, you're in it for life. But at least I've finally made it to the next level, and I am grateful.

"Let's take a vacation to celebrate this milestone," David suggests a few days later.

Over the years David and I have taken very few vacations together. Oh sure, we took various family vacations with the kids. We visited the Black Hills, Yellowstone, Glacier and other various national and state parks. We even splurged and took the "big trip" to Disney World, but we never ventured out too far or for too long as a couple. We had plenty of time to do that later, we told ourselves.

A cancer diagnosis changes perspective. This is what cancer does best; it changes things. We must no longer put off things like vacations because we don't really know how many more opportunities we will have for vacations, or for anything really. No one does, of course, but cancer delivers this message like a hard slap to the face.

"Where do you want to go?"

"How about Florida?" he asks.

Well of course it has to be someplace warm, though come to think of it, we have often traveled further north for vacations too. On the other hand, a warm destination would mean wearing less clothing and, God forbid, maybe even a swimsuit. I am afraid of swimsuits, and I'm pretty sure I'm not alone in this fear. Putting on a swimsuit can be a frightening thought for any woman. Throw in the pressure of wearing one after a bilateral mastectomy, even with reconstruction, and the idea takes on a whole new fear factor. But Florida it is. Me wearing a swimsuit, so be it.

One of the best things about being a cancer patient (and wearing a swimsuit for that matter) on vacation is that it's like traveling incognito; no one knows anything about you, including the fact that you've been dealing with cancer. This fact is wonderfully freeing. I walk down the street and feel normal, well, almost normal. People passing by have no idea who I am or what I've been through. I don't have to explain myself to anyone. I don't have to worry about my sparse crop of hair or about wearing a cap constantly. No one knows I recently finished chemotherapy. No one knows my genes are tainted. No one knows my breasts aren't really mine and that they have no nipples. No one knows I am facing more surgeries when I get home. No one knows I am still sometimes fearful and anxious. No one knows anything about me, and this makes me feel happier than I have felt in a long time.

"I feel like we are participants in some sort of witness protection program," I tell David.

I mention this while we take our daily walk along the beach feeling especially inconspicuous beneath my hat and dark sunglasses.

"What was the crime you witnessed?" he asks.

He knows the answer, but plays along, asking anyway.

"Cancer of course," I say.

"Of course."

"And I feel so ordinary, so average," I add.

Being average never felt so good. But vacation and feeling average end too soon. Too soon it's time to go home and face yet *more* surgery. Ugh...

Still, a vacation from myself was just what I needed, and it was fun while it lasted.

-40-

Another Hurdle

I am so not in a good place right now. I admit it. I am feeling quite grumpy and uncooperative. I feel like I am sitting poolside, but the pool I am sitting by is the one called the pool of self-pity. One little nudge and I'll fall completely in and will undoubtedly begin floundering and flailing around trying to figure out how not to drown.

I may have made it to the next level, but this level isn't all that great either. Being at this level means more female parts must go. How much of my femaleness do I have to sacrifice to this damn disease anyway? I didn't think this part would be quite so sucky, but it is. And tonight I have yet another meltdown.

"What is wrong with you?" David asks.

So much for spending a quiet evening watching TV. He looks me over trying to figure out what is wrong this time.

"I'm processing," I explain. "Crying is part of my processing."

He should know this about me by now shouldn't he?

"Facing yet another surgery is hard. Having more of my body parts yanked out, especially when there's nothing wrong with them, is in some ways even harder than when I removed both breasts."

"I had no idea you felt this way," he says.

Another reminder our loved ones are not mind readers.

It's time for another big moment on this hideous path I've been on for almost a year now. It's time for, yes, more surgery. It's time for my bilateral salpingo oophorectomy and total laparoscopic hyster-

179

ectomy. It's quite a mouthful even to say; the very words sound unpleasant.

This particular surgery will be of the assembly line variety. My doctors call it tag surgery, which really just means more than one surgeon is doing things. I like my assembly line description better. After surgeon number one finishes up, surgeon number two will be stepping in to complete a few finishing touches on my reconstruction project. Yep, it's time to create some fake nipples. The fun just never ends.

I have consulted five doctors about this particular hurdle and they all concurred. This hurdle is the recommended course of action due to my BRCA2 positive status. So why is coming to terms with this particular surgery so damn difficult? Wouldn't you think surgery impacting your inner organs would be less traumatic than, say, a bilateral mastectomy? Maybe, but then again, maybe not.

Deciding on my bilateral was "easy." There was a tumor involved, after all. It had to go. I am BRCA2 positive so both breasts had to go as well. Once I knew I was parting with one it was relatively "easy" to say goodbye to breast number two. Preparing for this surgery seems harder in some ways. My ovaries and uterus, too, are coming out only because they represent potential trouble. They might be too receptive to new cancer cell growth sometime in the future. The key word here is *might*. They *might* be troublemakers sometime down the road. Right now these organs are fine. This makes saying goodbye to them harder in a way. I have a whole new respect for all those women choosing prophylactic mastectomies and oophorectomies. They are making some tough, tough choices.

Perhaps another reason accepting this surgery is hard is because these organs represent fertility and femininity, and even though I'm done with the fertility part, my mind isn't. After all, the mind is a powerful force to be reckoned with. Or is it because it feels a bit like tempting fate? If something's not wrong, don't mess with it. Or is it hard because I'm soon facing the anniversary of my diagnosis? There are many heavily weighted dates looming. Did I plan poorly? Should I have waited longer? My oncologist doesn't believe in waiting here, this would be tempting fate of another kind. Is there a better time? And when might that be? I'm not sure, but I don't think there is. So…

I guess this is one more thing I must do. I must listen to my medical team. I must put my trust in them; I don't want to have regrets later. I want to get on with life and put this surgery, too, behind me. It's just one more hurdle.

Still, I can't help asking, how much does cancer have to take from me? How many body parts must I give up? How many times and in how many ways can one body be carved up? Sometimes I feel like I am not even myself anymore. Sometimes I feel as if I am no longer a woman at all. I am Frankenstein-like. Or maybe like Wonder Woman. Or the Bionic Woman. I am a reconstructed version of my former self, some sort of salvage job. But of course, in all the ways that matter I am still me. Or am I? I sure don't feel like it sometimes. How many hurdles do I still have to make it over? Perhaps it's better not to know.

It's time to hobble over this hurdle, too, and so I will. But it still pisses me off. A lot. And I have decided I am entitled to feel this way. Cancer is a string of losses, and there should be no shame in grieving for things lost and missed, including body parts. I am allowed. Damn it, I am allowed.

-41-

That Empty Space

When I travel back to Minnesota now to visit my dad, my parents' house feels like his house. It took me a while to get to this point, the point where visiting him isn't so incredibly sad because my mother is no longer there to visit too. For quite a while after my mother died, just walking around in their house or in the yard was really hard, really sad and made me physically and emotionally upset. My mother's presence was gone but at the same time it was everywhere. I could actually feel it. I guess I have finally made good progress on figuring out, or rather, adjusting to being a daughter without a mother in the physical sense.

Visits with my dad are pleasant, of course, but they are now filled with considerably less fanfare than when my mother was in charge. When our visits end, goodbyes are different now too.

My mother was the "Queen of Goodbyes." She perfected the simple act of saying goodbye following every visit into an art form. Saying goodbye after a visit was something that could never be ignored or hurried. She purposely made goodbyes a lengthy process in order to extend our visits as much as possible.

It didn't matter if I had come home for an hour visit, a day visit or a week-long visit. It didn't matter if I had just seen her the day before or if I would be back the next day. No matter the circumstance or length of my visit, when I left there was always a lengthy goodbye that could not be skipped or hurried.

First, there would be a hug in the doorway as I was getting ready to leave. Then we would proceed onto the front porch for more send-off hugs and last words. We never really used that front porch much when I was growing up. It faced the west side of the house, so the afternoon sun made it too hot to sit out there. And we always had dogs, so it was just easier to stay in the backyard, especially after it was fenced. So that porch became the porch of goodbyes, the place where my mother and I ended our visits and said goodbye.

Many times when I stepped off the porch of goodbyes, I also balanced paper plates piled with leftovers covered with foil Mother insisted on sending while I also juggled my purse, suitcase and whatever other belongings I had brought. It would have been simpler to just make a couple trips to the car but for some reason I always tried to get it all in one, miscalculating the amount of stuff I had brought home or accumulated during my visit. Mother always escorted me to my vehicle, and after I got inside, I lowered the window in order to do more waving and smiling as I backed out of the driveway. It had to be a pretty frigid day to keep her inside, and even then she stood in the doorway holding it wide open, waving me off as if I would not be seen again for years. My dad would undoubtedly comment about not wanting to "heat the outdoors," but it didn't matter and he knew it. He still felt obligated to say that. The door never closed until I had turned the corner and was out of sight. Warm days enabled our goodbyes to be lengthier and more pleasant; we could linger even longer.

I have often wondered if goodbyes in other families are such a production. I know my mother learned it from her mother. I can still picture my grandma wearing her green, knit pants and perfectly ironed blouse with tiny flowers printed on it, standing alone on her driveway in her low-heeled, beige, leather shoes waving goodbye at the end of a summer visit. I don't picture my grandpa out there. He usually slipped me and my siblings each a ten-dollar bill, gave us a hug and sent us on our way. Is it easier for men to say goodbye? Or are they simply quieter about it?

I never gave much thought to what my final goodbye to Mother might be like. In a way this is odd since I always knew how important goodbyes were to her. Perhaps I just didn't want to think about that day. Perhaps I was afraid to imagine how my life would change when I became motherless. Maybe I should've thought about these things.

Maybe all daughters should.

These days when I visit my dad, one thing I can't help but notice is our goodbyes are much quicker now. Another thing I notice is this goodbye time is a time I really miss my mother; I always will. I miss those long goodbyes she loved so much.

Even now when I get into my car and pull out of the driveway, I still expect to see my mother standing there on the front porch or on the driveway waving as I drive off. Instead, all I see is that empty space where she is supposed to be standing.

It's often the simple things you miss the most about your loved ones when they are gone. It doesn't even have to be something tangible. It might be their scent. It might be a particular mannerism. It might be a certain expression. It might be their laugh. It might be the way their presence filled up a room. Or it might be the way they said goodbye.

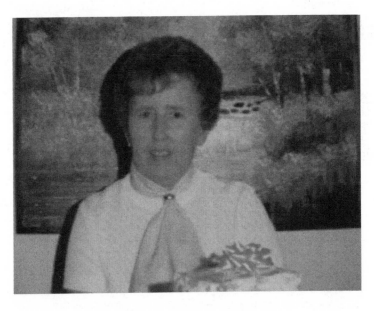

My mother, our "Queen of Goodbyes"

-42-

Moving Forward

It's been more than a year since my diagnosis, so it's time to start taking stock of things, or so I'm told. I'm supposed to be making good progress on picking up the pieces. I'm supposed to start putting cancer behind me and find my "new normal," whatever that means. And how do you do this when you have no clue as to how to go about it and when you know darn well the cancer cloud will be forever hovering? It's interesting how this applies to both grieving for my mother and to my cancer experience. Society seems to be nudging, no, more like pushing me, to hurry up. Be done. Put them behind me. Move on. Forget about them. Get back to the way things were. These are the subtle messages. The trouble is, it's not quite that simple, or even possible. The truth is, I will never be done with either one. And guess what? I don't even want to be done.

Maybe you're sitting there reading this, asking, who in her right mind would not want to be done with grieving and cancer? But the way I see it, this would be like erasing parts of my life. It would be like denying I have brown eyes, three siblings, graduated from Madelia High School, taught second grade, am a happily married woman and have three amazing kids. I don't erase those parts of my life when I think about or describe myself. Breast cancer and loss experiences are now part of who I am, too, so how or why would I forget about them even if I could?

I am reminded every day when I look in the mirror that I'm much altered physically. The emotional scars aren't as obvious, but they are there as well, so I can't forget anyway. And yes, I miss my breasts. Sometimes it seems I'm not supposed to think or say this, much less state such a thing in a book. Even staring at those printed words seems strange. Stating them out loud feels stranger still. After all, I'm alive. Shouldn't this be enough? Well yes, but I still miss them.

In a way, having a mastectomy has almost become some weird kind of normal. It's not. Along with all the discussion about mastectomies these days, there is a lot of reconstruction talk as well. Sometimes this process is made to sound too easy, almost normal-like too. Again, it's not. Reconstruction is no free boob job and reconstructed breasts may or may not turn out lovely, but regardless, they are still reconstructed. They are still stand-ins for the real deal, a salvage job at best. When I'm fully clothed after my reconstruction, no one can tell by looking at me I am not the same as before. *But I can tell. I know.* Reconstruction is a cosmetic "fix" at best. And if a woman chooses not to do reconstruction, she might be looked upon with skepticism, perhaps even made to feel she must explain her reasons for opting out and making the "radical" choice she did. None of this is in any way normal-like, easy or easily forgotten.

In addition to the physical and emotional scars after a breast cancer diagnosis, there are all the nasty, long-term and lingering side effects from treatment too numerous to list. And let's not forget the most awful lingering "side effect" of all, living the rest of your life knowing cancer can reappear any time down the road. So it's not really even possible to file away your cancer experience as "finished." Cancer is never that tidy. Cancer is never over. Grief isn't either.

I have learned I am allowed to feel loss and gratitude at the same time. I do have much to be grateful for and I am, but I also have things and people to grieve for and miss because cancer changes everything and impacts just about every aspect of your life. And despite how things are often depicted in the media and in Pink Ribbon Fantasy Land, nothing about any of it is easy or easily forgotten. Cancer is not just a bump in the road. If there is one thing in life that definitely fits that "game-changer" cliché, cancer just might be it.

Not forgetting does not mean I am stuck in Cancer Land or that I am unable to move forward. I am not and I do. However, I will do it in my own time and in my own way. I feel quite strongly about this; I am not finished with cancer or grieving. There is more to process, more to do and so much more to share about both.

Survivorship warrants another whole book of its own anyway. This part of the cancer experience isn't easy either. In fact, it's damn hard due to a whole variety of reasons. A main one is because no one prepares you. If you're one of the "lucky" ones and able to finish up active cancer treatment, you're more or less turned loose and sent on your merry way to figure things out on your own.

On top of heading into survivorship unprepared, once you land in this new and unchartered territory, you are once again inundated with far too many outside pressures and expectations about how to do this part of cancer too. The advice regarding finding that elusive "new normal" starts rolling in and can seem never ending. It's sometimes helpful but often not. Some embrace the "new normal" concept. Others resist. As for me, I have not figured out how anything cancer related can have any kind of normalcy to it, new or otherwise. Nothing about cancer is normal. Nothing about survivorship is either; I am still tip-toeing through it.

After a certain amount of time passes in your post-cancer-diagnosis life (regardless of stage), society tells you you're supposed to have learned some things and morphed into a new and improved version of your former self. This feels like one more "cancer obligation" you're supposed to fulfill. Cancer does not miraculously make you a better person, or a worse one for that matter.

And here's the real stunner for me. There is pressure out there to view your cancer experience as a positive thing, perhaps even to consider it to be something you are grateful to have gone through. *Some go so far as to call cancer the best thing that ever happened to them, a gift even.* Do you hear the fingernails on the chalkboard yet?

Calling cancer a gift or an "opportunity" for personal enlightenment makes a nice feature story for a magazine or newspaper article, but it's not reality, at least it's not mine. Plus, it's downright insulting to those with a stage IV diagnosis. Maybe it is just all semantics, but words matter. A lot. I will never be calling cancer a gift. People are gifts. Life is a gift. Cancer is not. This doesn't mean I am bitter, negative or ungrateful. Mostly, it means I'm a person who lives in reality.

If looking at their cancer as a gift works for some, more power to them. I mean that. But as for me, this kind of thinking is unfathomable. Cancer was not, is not and never will be a gift for me and my family. Despite the illusion created by pink ribbon culture, breast cancer is still a horrible, too often deadly disease, and nothing about it is pretty, pink or gift-like. Period.

No one should feel pressured to accomplish profound things following a cancer diagnosis either. No matter what your cancer stage, trying to reclaim and maintain your life and sanity will be profound enough. Trust me. You do not necessarily need to throw out all your old ways and drive yourself, your family or both nuts in the process. Make changes and improvements in your lifestyle choices, yes, but don't go crazy worrying about every little thing you do or do not do. Eat as healthy as you can, for sure. Exercise, yes, but don't beat yourself up trying to run marathons or climb Mt. Kilimanjaro, unless of course, you want to. And you are not obligated to write a blog or a book, mentor others, walk or run in races, deck yourself out in pink, start a foundation or whatever it is you think you're supposed to do now. You don't have to do any of that stuff. Just getting back to living your life is a huge deal and more than enough to figure out.

No matter what stage you were diagnosed at or where you are in treatment, figuring out your life post diagnosis will keep you plenty busy. And there is only one way for you to do it—your way. Don't allow anyone to tell you anything different. So ditch the pressures and expectations. Who needs them? I wish someone had given me this little piece of advice at the start of my cancer maze. Maybe I had to figure it out for myself. Maybe we all do, but by sharing, perhaps we can save each other some time and minimize some of the frustration.

For a lot of reasons, cancer will never be over for me. I am moving forward, still slowly at times, but this is okay. Somehow, in my mind anyway, moving forward is different than moving on. Moving on seems to imply you should move on and leave the past tucked neatly behind you. I prefer to think of myself as moving forward while taking my cancer experience, and all the others (the good and the bad), with me. It's the same with my grief. I don't move on and leave my mother behind. I move forward taking her with me in my heart. I move forward a changed person but still the same too.

Maybe this really just means I was flawed and not finished evolving before cancer, and I am flawed and not finished evolving today. I was just me. I am still just me. I will always be just me. And this is enough.

Afterword

At the time of this book's publishing, I am five years post cancer diagnosis. I am still picking up the pieces and trying to figure out this thing called survivorship. It has taken me five years to organize my thoughts, finish this part of my story and get it out there. The time finally feels right, and I am ready to share it. I know there are many cancer stories out there and I am sharing yet another, but there is room for all our stories. I fully realize many people are not comfortable with or interested in reading or talking about cancer realities, much less death, grief and loss. I hope by sharing my story about these things, I am playing a small role in helping to change this. We should talk about cancer realities. We should talk about dying. We should talk about death. We should talk about grief. We should talk about these things even if it's hard, maybe because it's hard.

After five years, I am still NED (no evidence of disease) and for this I am grateful every day. Many of my friends are not so lucky, and this is one more reason I will never be calling cancer a gift. It's not. How can something be a gift for me and at the same time be the reason for someone else's suffering and death? How could something that killed my own mother ever be considered something good that happened to me?

Each year in the United States alone, roughly 40,000 women and men still die from metastatic breast cancer. Sadly, many people are unaware of this statistic because the messages put out by the Pink Machine too often do not share this information. Early detection is important, but it is not the whole story. And the whole story matters. It always does. Some cancers will metastasize regardless of what stage they are diagnosed at. Some cancers are diagnosed initially as stage IV, and no, this does not mean the person did anything wrong. This stigma has to end. We must continue to educate about the entire spectrum of this disease because *breast cancer awareness without metastatic awareness isn't awareness at all.*

Cancer has brought many changes into my life, some of them good, most of them not. I have learned some things along the way, some of it good, much of it not. Two things I still believe to be true are: *cancer was not a gift and it didn't make me a better person.*

189

About the Author

Nancy Stordahl is a former educator and now a freelance writer and blogger. She was raised in Minnesota and currently resides in Wisconsin with her husband and pets. She has three grown children. To contact, visit www.NancysPoint.com.

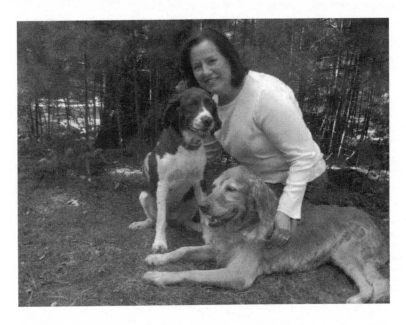

The author with Sophie and Elsie, her two special grief and cancer eyewitnesses and secret keepers. Elsie died from cancer in August 2015, loyal companion to the end.

Cancer is not a ribbon, a screening test or a leisure activity. It is not a sassy t-shirt, a proclamation of survivorship or a gift worth giving. It is a disease process that ignites what is all too often a cycle of medical surveillance and interventions, of which some succeed and others cause irreparable harm. For too many, it will be the eventual cause of death. They deserve better than this, and so do we.

Gayle A. Sulik, Ph.D.

A note from the author about the cover

I always knew my book's cover would have no pink ribbons. I also knew I wanted it to have special meaning. This is why I chose to have an image from www.NancysPoint.com on the cover. It reminds me of my dear readers. It reminds me of my favorite season. It reminds me of nature's beauty. It reminds me of life. These are gifts. Cancer is not.

Made in the USA
Middletown, DE
02 November 2017